The Researching Therapist

For Churchill Livingstone:

Editorial Director: Mary Law
Project Manager: Valerie Burgess
Project Editor: Dinah Thom
Copy Editor: Jennifer Bew
Indexer: Tarrant Ranger Indexing Agency
Design Direction: Judith Wright
Sales Promotion Executive: Hilary Brown

The Researching Therapist

A Practical Guide to Planning, Performing and Communicating Research

Sue Jenkins DipPhys PhD
Senior Lecturer, Cardiopulmonary Program Coordinator,
School of Physiotherapy, Curtin University of Technology, Perth, Western Australia

Connie J Price BSPE BScPT MSc PhD
Physical Therapist, and Special Projects Officer, Royal Perth Hospital
and Lecturer, School of Physiotherapy, Curtin University of Technology, Perth, Western Australia

Leon Straker BSc(Physio) MSc PhD
Senior Lecturer, Ergonomics Program Coordinator, School of Physiotherapy,
Curtin University of Technology, Perth, Western Australia

Foreword by

Lance T. Twomey AM BAppSc BSc PhD
Vice-Chancellor and Professor, Curtin University of Technology,
Perth, Western Australia

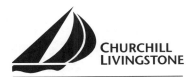

CHURCHILL LIVINGSTONE

NEW YORK EDINBURGH LONDON MADRID MELBOURNE SAN FRANCISCO TOKYO 1998

CHURCHILL LIVINGSTONE
Medical Division of Pearson Professional Limited

Distributed in the United States of America by Churchill Livingstone, 650 Avenue of the Americas, New York, N.Y. 10011, and by associated companies, branches and representatives throughout the world.

© Pearson Professional Limited 1998

⬧ is a registered trademark of Pearson Professional Limited.

First published 1998

ISBN 0443 057613

British Library Cataloguing in Publication Data
A catalogue record for this book is available from the British Library.

Library of Congress Cataloging in Publication Data
A catalog record for this book is available from the Library of Congress.

Note
Medical knowledge is constantly changing. As new information becomes available, changes in treatment, procedures, equipment and the use of drugs become necessary. The authors and the publishers have, as far as it is possible, taken care to ensure that the information given in this text is accurate and up-to-date. However, readers are strongly advised to confirm that the information, especially with regard to drug usage, complies with latest legislation and standards of practice.

The publisher's policy is to use **paper manufactured from sustainable forests**

Produced through Longman Malaysia, PP

Contents

Acknowledgements

We would like to thank the following for their valuable contributions to the book, especially in ensuring that it encompassed speech, occupational and physical therapies, and the various qualitative and quantitative approaches to research used within these therapies:

Vaile Drake DipOT PGDiP HlthSc MSc
Lecturer, School of Occupational Therapy, Curtin University of Technology, Perth, Western Australia

Neville Hennessey BA(Hons) PhD
Lecturer, School of Speech and Hearing Science, Curtin University of Technology, Perth, Western Australia

Rick Ladyshewsky BMedRehab MHlthScAdmin
Lecturer, School of Physiotherapy, Curtin University of Technology, Perth, Western Australia

Cathy Robertson BST(Hons)
Lecturer, School of Speech and Hearing Science, Curtin University of Technology, Perth, Western Australia

Kevin Singer DipPT DipTch MSc PhD
Associate Professor, School of Physiotherapy, Curtin University of Technology, Perth, Western Australia

Foreword

The disciplines of occupational therapy, physiotherapy and speech pathology have always been recognized as superb practical professions, which have gone from strength to strength throughout the 20th century. This is attested by the quality of their entering students and by the more central role they have progressively assumed in diagnosis and treatment worldwide. Their practitioners have always been proud of their practical skills, their ability to get down to work and the regard in which they are held by their clients. Although these attributes remain important, health services and governments are now demanding a higher level of proof of efficacy, cost-effectiveness and performance. In most instances this is difficult, if not impossible, to provide, as the theory base for the therapy professions has been shown to be more strongly anecdotal than centred on science and backed by the evidence of sound research. These disciplines have for too long neglected science and scholarship and have too highly regarded ephemeral praise from grateful patients.

Although the volume of applied research in the therapies has increased very considerably over the last decade, because it started from an almost zero base it still does not amount to a substantial body of work in any of their many subdisciplines. It is certainly time for these professions to address the situation and to strongly support and better value the development of a substantial body of scholarship.

The current emphasis on postgraduate education has encouraged research and resulted in a considerable increase in the 'scientific content' of the journals in all therapy disciplines. There has been reaction to this new emphasis from some practitioners, who view such activity as esoteric and too removed from the 'real world' of patients and their problems.

However, few practitioners are in a position to really know whether the treatments they so enthusiastically support are truly effective. Indeed, many recent studies have cast substantial doubt on time-honoured treatment practices.

It is certainly time for there to be an even greater focus on research in the therapies. It is not too dramatic to state that the long-term future of the professions rests on the ability of their practitioners to justify established techniques and practices and to establish cost-efficiency. In this regard, schools of occupational therapy, physiotherapy and speech pathology, and the scholarship they engender, are central to the initiative. This book fills an important niche, in that it guides the beginning researching therapist through the process of research in a down-to-earth, practical manner. It integrates quantitative and qualitative research with excellent applied examples, and provides information on the important topics associated with scholarship.

Ethical situations, the authorship of papers, collaborative research, the student/supervisor relationship and the like are effectively covered within this volume. This is an excellent book which will provide strong support to those therapists who wish to be at the forefront of their professions in the next millennium.

L.T.

Preface

The aim of this book is to guide the researching therapist through the processes involved with research, processes which to the new or inexperienced researcher are often bewildering and intimidating. The book is intended for use by practising therapists wishing to evaluate aspects of their clinical practice, and for students in the allied health disciplines undertaking research at all levels, from undergraduate to doctoral studies. This is a generic book written for therapists from the occupational therapy, physiotherapy and speech pathology disciplines and, although aimed at the researching therapist, it will also be of use to supervisors and reviewers of research. The book has been written with research in mind; however, the information in some chapters – for example relating to writing in scientific style and presenting research – will be useful to therapists in other aspects of professional life. In preparing the book the authors have drawn on their experiences as practising therapists and researchers, and experience acquired through the supervision of researching therapists.

The structure of the book is such that it follows the research process from the identification of a problem to the communication of findings; however, the material is organized to enable an immediate need for specific information to be met by reading individual chapters in isolation. To assist with the assimilation of information, examples from occupational therapy, physiotherapy and speech therapy have been included. Key points, and common errors and misconceptions encountered by researach supervisors, have been identified throughout the book and are presented in 'Key Points' and 'Hazard' boxes, respectively. The 'Further Reading' box at the end of each chapter directs the reader to additional material.

The text is divided into four main sections:

- Section 1 provides an introduction to the research process.
- Section 2 deals with planning for research. The chapters in this section consider the different stages involved, from the selection of a research topic through to the writing and presenting of a research proposal. The final chapters discuss planning for ethical research and provide the researching therapist with information to increase the likelihood of success when applying for research funding.
- Section 3 is concerned with performing research and considers the effective use of resources and the issue of managing data and controlling quality.
- Section 4 begins by discussing the need communicate research findings. Subsequent chapters aim to assist the researching therapist with the development of a high standard of communication skills. Individual chapters deal with the writing of a thesis and a journal article. A prerequisite for written research communications is the use of a scientific writing style and the appropriate use of clear figures and tables; separate chapters are devoted to these topics. Section 4 concludes with chapters relating to the scientific conference and discusses how to make the most of conference attendance.

The appendices provide useful examples of data collection sheets and informed consent documents, and includes a section on typography.

S.J., C.P. & L.S.   Perth 1997

1 Introduction

SECTION CONTENTS

The research process

This chapter argues the need for therapists to be involved in research. A model of the research process is presented and the components of the process briefly described, with cross-references to the chapters in this book which provide details on each component.

THE NEED FOR RESEARCH BY THE THERAPIES

Many therapies have a tradition of authority-based practice dogma. Whereas this may have been adequate in the past, changes in the expectations of consumers, professional colleagues and funding organizations now require a more rigorous validation of clinical practices. Therefore, a major challenge facing these professions is not only to provide high-quality patient management but also to be able to substantiate the quality, efficacy and efficiency of that management. High-quality research to provide substantial and convincing evidence to support the claims of optimal patient management has been lacking, and is thus urgently required.

Fortunately, the increase in accountability requirements of the professions has been paralleled by the development of a large body of research methods. These are commonly grouped into two main types: experimental/positivistic/quantitative, and naturalistic/interpretive/qualitative. Although there are some researchers who criticize quantitative and others who criticize qualitative, both types are essential to the development of the body of knowledge required by the therapies. Neither type is capable of adequately providing all the answers to the questions therapists ask. Therapists should therefore use whichever type is most appropriate for answering a question.

Although the need for research to provide the evidence to justify clinical practices is acknowledged by most therapists, for those without research experience the thought of performing research can be intimidating. Fear of the unknown probably contributes to the unwillingness of some therapists to perform research. This book aims to alleviate this fear by describing the practicalities of completing a research project. The following section introduces and describes a model of research which is used as the structure for this book.

A MODEL OF THE RESEARCH PROCESS

The aim of research is to increase knowledge. Hence each individual research project can be thought of as a small circle spinning off a continuum of knowledge. The project begins from the current knowledge base, and should eventually contribute back to that knowledge base, as illustrated in Figure 1.1.

Each project cycle must complete three stages: planning for research, performing research and communicating the research findings (Fig. 1.2). Without any one of these stages the research process would not be complete.

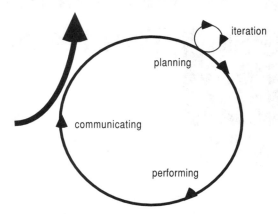

Figure 1.2 Representation of the three stages of a research project

Within each stage a number of components will need to be completed, though the exact components will vary depending on the type of research. There may also be iteration, especially in the planning phase. For example, the initial research question selected may be found to be unsuitable after development and the researching therapist would return to select another question, as represented in the small iteration circle in Figure 1.2. The remainder of this chapter provides a brief description of common components within each of the three stages, and thus provides an overview of the following chapters in this book.

Components of the planning stage

The research planning stage can be considered to involve the following: choosing a research question, evaluating research resources, developing a research question, writing a research proposal, presenting the research proposal, planning for ethical research and applying for research funding.

Choosing a research question

Selecting an interesting and original research question or topic takes a surprising amount of time. Research begins as a query, often stimulated by curiosity, and leads to a quest for an answer. The process of choosing the research question is

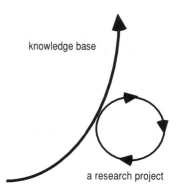

Figure 1.1 Representation of an individual research project developing from and returning to the knowledge base

expanded in Chapter 2, which suggests that the researching therapist should develop a list of possible research questions. These should then be evaluated against a number of criteria, which include the available resources.

Evaluating research resources

Chapter 3 argues that the researcher should review the available resources before determining a workable research question. The therapist must consider their competence to undertake the research process according to their knowledge, capabilities and limitations, and their reasons for wishing to undertake research. Other important considerations include access to literature and other research resources, such as subjects, experts in areas where the researcher lacks specialist skills, access to equipment and facilities and, if necessary, funding.

Developing a research question

Once a research question has been selected it should be developed by identifying the most appropriate type of research, defining the main terms in the question, declaring the assumptions, biases and perspectives, and identifying limitations. The development of a research question usually also involves refining a broad problem down to specific guiding questions or hypotheses, as described in Chapter 4.

Writing a research proposal

Writing a research proposal is a critical part of planning for research, as it documents the plan for performing the research. Chapter 5 outlines the purpose of the research proposal and details the structure and content of a typical proposal. The proposal represents the first opportunity for the prospective researcher to demonstrate their ability to integrate information from different sources and articulate a research plan. Writing the research proposal also gives the researching therapist a sense of accomplishment at having passed the first major milestone.

Presenting the research proposal

Presenting the research proposal allows vital peer review of the research plan prior to implementation. The research question should be clearly articulated, together with the details of how data will be collected to answer the question. This process, described in Chapter 6, allows for fine tuning and modification of the study design to accommodate useful suggestions which might not have been considered. This emphasizes the point that good research benefits from wide exposure of ideas to colleagues before the study is implemented. This helps to ensure that the project has value and is able to answer the research question.

Planning for ethical research

Obtaining appropriate ethical clearance for the project is a mandatory requirement of most research. The process ensures that all checks have been performed and the study has been affirmed for scientific as well as ethical standards. A detailed summary of the ethical review process is provided in Chapter 7.

Applying for funding

Funding is often desired or essential to enable a research project to be performed. Chapter 8 uses the analogy of the futures market to explain the process of applying for research funding.

Components of the performing stage

After adequate planning, the researching therapist is ready to carry out the research project. Performing research requires that the research therapist be able to work as part of a team, to seek out and use the advice of experts, to manage time wisely and to undertake processes for managing data and controlling quality.

Working as part of a team

Many research projects involve a team of researchers. As with any team endeavour, the team needs to work well together for the project to be performed effectively. Chapter 9 provides guidelines to assist the researching therapist in establishing and maintaining good team relations.

Using experts

Experts in research design, methods and analysis, clinical experts and project management experts are among those commonly needed by the researching therapist. Suggestions on effective use of these important resources are given in Chapter 10.

Using time wisely

Time is perhaps one's most valuable resource, yet many therapists could improve their management of time. Chapter 11 discusses mechanisms to help the researching therapist use time wisely, to allow time for the other things in life and to enable the research project to be completed to plan.

Managing data and controlling quality

During the performance of research stage the goal is to collect data to answer the research question. It is therefore of vital importance to the trustworthiness of the answer that data are carefully managed as they are collected, and that quality is thoroughly controlled. Chapter 12 describes practical methods to ensure that data are of high quality.

Components of the communicating stage

Having performed a research project, the researching therapist has a responsibility to communicate their findings to peers and to the community, and thus contribute back to the knowledge base. The components of the final stage of research may include: communicating research; writing in scientific style; preparing graphs, tables and other figures; dealing with authorship; writing a thesis; writing a journal article; presenting research; attending a scientific conference; preparing a conference poster; and chairing a session at a conference.

Communicating research

Chapter 13 provides an introduction to the final stage of research by discussing the various types of research communication and the importance of communicating research findings competently.

Writing in scientific style

An important aspect of successful communication is the ability to produce written material which is clear and unambiguous. Chapter 14 presents detailed guidelines to assist the researching therapist develop the skill of concise but informative written communication.

Preparing graphs, tables and other figures

A second important means of communicating research information is through competent use of graphs, tables and other figures. Many researching therapists will have experienced the frustration of trying to interpret information presented in an inappropriate or poorly designed figure or table. Although the design of figures and tables can be complex, Chapter 15 provides an understanding of the different types and their various uses. The chapter includes suggestions for which type of figure or table to use, and how to design them for effective communication.

Dealing with authorship

One of the issues that can lead to a breakdown in effective communication of research findings is that of authorship. Chapter 16 outlines the potential problems and suggests ways of negotiating suitable agreements on authorship.

Writing a thesis

For some researching therapists, their second major written communication (after the proposal) is the thesis. Writing a well structured and informative thesis is often thought to be the most difficult research task. Chapter 17 provides information to make this process much easier. One of the dilemmas often faced is how to structure the thesis, and Chapter 17 includes a number of examples suitable for a wide range of research designs. Details of the content expected in each section are given, together with information on the examination process and thesis defence.

Writing a journal article

The most effective and permanent means of communicating research findings to peers is by publication of an article in a widely indexed, peer-reviewed journal. The processes of choosing a suitable journal, preparing a manuscript with suitable structure and content, submitting the manuscript and dealing with comments from the editor and reviewer are outlined in Chapter 18.

Presenting research

Another popular method of communicating research findings is by verbal presentation at a conference. Chapter 19 describes the preparation of the structure, content and audiovisual aids for a verbal presentation, with particular reference to conferences.

Attending a scientific conference

Communication of research information occurs not only via journal articles but also by participation at a scientific conference. Chapter 20 suggests how to choose a suitable conference and how to maximize the opportunities conference attendance provides. Details on the preparation of a poster for a conference are provided in Chapter 21, and Chapter 22 discusses another opportunity for research communication, chairing a session at a conference.

The research process typically involves developing a research question and a method for answering that question, performing the research to provide the data to answer the question, and communicating the findings back to peers and the wider community. The need for therapists to become researchers is clear. This book provides the guidance to allow therapists to become competent researchers able to provide substantial and convincing evidence to support the claims of optimal patient management.

Further Reading

Findley T W, Daum M C, Stineman M 1990 Research in physical medicine VII: the principal investigator. American Journal of Physical Medicine Rehabilitation 69: 39–45

Hulley S B, Cummings S R 1988 Designing clinical research. Williams & Wilkins, Baltimore

Leedy P D 1993 Practical research: planning and design, 5th edn. McMillan, New York

Marshall C, Rossman G B 1995 Designing qualitative research, 2nd edn. Sage, Thousand Oaks

2

Planning for research

SECTION CONTENTS

2 Choosing a research question

This chapter is intended to assist a researching therapist to choose a suitable research question. A model of how to do this is introduced and the various elements of the model are described.

According to Payton (1988), research is the process of seeking an answer to a question in an organized and consistent way. Asking a question is thus the first step. Choosing the right question to ask is perhaps the most important part of the research process, as it directs all subsequent planning and analysis. The research question usually starts as a broad, diffuse question which is later developed into a researchable one (see Chapter 4).

However, choosing a suitable question is not necessarily an easy task, and making poor choices at this stage can result in a frustrating experience in which the considerable effort invested seems futile. To help avoid such frustration, this chapter provides a model for the researching therapist to follow to choose a question which will be researchable and relevant. Figure 2.1 shows the model and its four main elements: 1) the analysis of the current situation, 2) the generation of possible research questions, 3) the evaluation of possible research questions and 4) the selection of a priority research question. Details of these elements are provided in the sections that follow.

ANALYSE CURRENT SITUATION

An analysis of the current situation involves gathering information about the researching

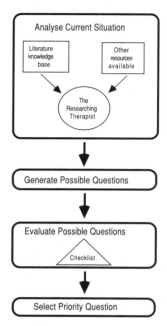

Figure 2.1 A model of how to choose a research question

therapist's capabilities, limitations and goals, the literature base and the other resources available. A knowledge of the resources available will guide the researching therapist to what is possible, including which types of research are suitable. Chapter 3 describes these resources in detail. Once the current situation has been thoroughly analysed, it is appropriate to generate some possible research questions.

GENERATE POSSIBLE RESEARCH QUESTIONS

New researchers are sometimes overawed by the prospect of generating a research question. However, this is often because it is thought that the first question generated must be the most appropriate. The model described here makes generating research questions easier, as it suggests that questions generated at this stage need only be *possible* questions.

Most working therapists will be able to 'brain-storm' numerous possible research questions. Situations which may prompt questions include clinical practice, professional meetings, professional reading, and discussions with colleagues, students and patients.

During clinical practice phenomena may be evident which are hard to understand or define, or it may become apparent that valid and reliable assessment tools need to be developed or refined, or that prevailing beliefs are limiting treatment options, all of which suggest potential research topics. Research presented at a conference, special interest group or departmental meeting may challenge assumptions currently held by the therapist. In addition, most research reports contain recommendations for further study. Verbal presentations of research findings and written research reports may stimulate a desire to replicate a study to verify the success or failure of a treatment, or to show inconsistencies or limitations which require further study. Descriptive case studies may also stimulate the generation of researchable questions.

Discussions with colleagues may highlight differences of opinion or shared interests for research. A therapist is often stimulated by the queries raised by students and clients to re-evaluate their knowledge base and identify weak areas requiring clarification. Recently, Internet discussion groups have been used to gather potential research questions from colleagues.

Some examples of possible research questions are given below:

- *How does a person's cultural background influence success in therapy?*
- *Do children with mild phonology disorders respond better to parent-provided therapy or direct intervention therapy by a clinician?*
- *Is eccentric muscle training able to produce more rapid strength and endurance gains for clients following a whiplash injury?*

As can be seen, the questions can be quite broad, depending on what is known in the area and the focus of the research. Once a number of possible questions have been generated they can be evaluated.

Key Point 2.1

Time should be allowed to evaluate possible research questions adequately

EVALUATE POSSIBLE RESEARCH QUESTIONS

The evaluation of possible research questions requires a comparison of each with the information gathered from the analysis of the current situation. Thus the possible questions are compared with the capabilities, limitations and goals of the researching therapist, the extent and nature of the literature, and the other resources available.

In addition, the question should be worthwhile, comply with employment or study requirements, allow for changes in the research environment, have data which can be collected to answer it, and be answerable with ethical research.

Research takes a considerable amount of time, thought and effort. It is something a researcher should be proud of. A commendable research topic should be both interesting and worthwhile: if the only response elicited from describing a potential research topic is 'So what?', perhaps the question is not significant enough to be worth the effort. To help judge the significance and relevance of the research topic it is useful to imagine the possible outcomes to clinical practice, scientific knowledge, clinical and health policy, and future research directions.

Researching therapists frequently conduct research either as part of postgraduate studies or as part of employment. Hence the particular requirements specified by the academic institution or employer need to be considered.

The therapist should also be cognisant of the clinical, political, social, cultural and industrial environment within which the research will be conducted. The therapist rarely has control over this environment once a study has begun, so careful consideration should be given to possible changes and their impact on the study outcome. For example, the clinical environment may change when the management of a certain client problem is shifted into community care rather than hospital care. Such a change would disrupt research on what it means to be hospitalized.

Potential changes in social attitudes and political power may create changes which hamper the ability of a therapist to continue to provide an intervention. A significant event given prominence by the media can rapidly polarize social attitudes and lead to political change. For example, a spate of violent crimes may give rise to community demands, and political action, for tougher parole management of criminals. This could have a devastating effect on a study investigating the effectiveness of a voluntary activity programme on recidivism rates and prisoner attitudes to society.

Similarly, the cultural setting may make certain types of investigations impossible. For example, some cultural groups do not permit disrobing. This would make accurate assessment and treatment of certain patient problems difficult. Thus attempts to use biofeedback to improve head stability in clients with poor eating ability using electromyography of the neck and jaw muscles may be impossible if the client group must maintain strict head coverage.

Some study designs require significant cooperation across industrial groups, which may be jeopardized by industrial relations difficulties. For instance, an occupational health intervention study which used the workers from multiple workplaces randomly allocated to interventions would be compromised if some of the workers went on strike during the study period. Not only would the workers not have been performing their normal duties, they might also have potentially important changes in attitudes to the workplace which could interact with the study's intervention.

For a research question to be suitable it should be feasible to collect information which will provide evidence for an answer. Pertinent data, alternatively called phenomena or variables, range from being easy to identify and collect (knee strength, wet weight of sputum expectorated, correctness of answers to a test) to being hard to describe, let alone identify (professionalism, non-verbal communication skills). Some phenomena are fairly easy to measure (height, weight, heart rate, reported importance of control over therapy), whereas others are very difficult (deep muscle electromyographic activity, dysphasia). To provide an adequate answer, the phenomena must be measurable. For example, a quantitative rehabilitation study where the question is 'How many clients return to productive life within the community following intervention X?' needs to determine what is productive. If no agreed meaning can be found then an appropriate research question may be 'What is the meaning of productive to clients?', and this could be well answered using a qualitative method.

Finally, the research topic should allow for an ethical research design. For many years tobacco companies have been able to claim that it is not proven that tobacco smoking causes lung cancer in humans, despite epidemiological correlations, biochemical studies and animal studies suggesting otherwise. To actually prove the causal relationship in humans one would have to conduct an experiment where one group of subjects was randomly allocated to tobacco use with cancer outcomes for this tobacco using group and a second control group monitored. However, given the strong and sufficient evidence (to everyone except tobacco company officials) that tobacco does cause cancer in humans, it would be unethical to conduct such a study.

To assist the new researcher with the process of evaluating potential research questions, an evaluation checklist has been devised (Table 2.1). It will also be useful to discuss ideas with 'friendly' experts, although care should be taken that a well resourced expert does not take the question and answer it before the researching therapist can complete the proposal! Also, care should be taken not to waste experts' time with ill-considered ideas. (Chapter 3 describes some of the important aspects of research resources in detail, and should be read prior to attempting to use the evaluation checklist.)

SELECT PRIORITY RESEARCH QUESTION

Following evaluation there is likely to be a small

Table 2.1 Research question evaluation checklist

	Rating		
Therapist	Low	Mid	High
Likely design suits personal traits?	*	*	*
Builds on current knowledge and skills?	*	*	*
Will further career and personal goals?	*	*	*
Question is of interest and excites?	*	*	*
Literature			
Reasonable literature base?	*	*	*
Recent literature interest in area?	*	*	*
Question unanswered in recent literature?	*	*	*
Other resources			
Suitable, willing subjects in adequate numbers available?	*	*	*
Required expertise available?	*	*	*
Required equipment, facilities, space available?	*	*	*
Timescale appropriate?	*	*	*
Reasonable potential for funding if needed?	*	*	*
Additional questions			
Is the question significant?	*	*	*
Will employer/academic requirements be met?	*	*	*
Changes in research environment unlikely to stop research?	*	*	*
Able to collect data to answer question?	*	*	*
Likely design ethical?	*	*	*
Overall rating	*	*	*

group of research questions which were rated favourably. The single question which is most likely to meet the needs of the current situation should then be selected. Critically, given the necessary time and energy investment, the question should be satisfying to the researching therapist.

Hazard 2.1

Settling on the first question which stimulates interest

Unable to generate a research question owing to thinking the first question must be perfect

Although the model of how to choose a research question has been presented in a purely linear form, in most cases it is iterative. Thus initial questions may be found to be unsuitable and a new group of possible questions will need to be generated and evaluated. One of the most important aspects of the process is the review of resources, which Chapter 3 reviews in detail.

REFERENCE

Payton O D 1988 Research: the validation of clinical practice, 2nd edn. F A Davis, Philadelphia

Evaluating research resources

As outlined in Chapter 2, a thorough evaluation of the resources available to the researching therapist will facilitate the choice of a practicable and feasible research topic. These resources can be divided into three categories: personal resources, the literature base and other research resources. This chapter discusses the most important aspects of each of these categories.

THERAPIST'S CAPABILITIES, LIMITATIONS AND GOALS

The personal resources of the researching therapist include their traits, work experience and areas of expertise, research knowledge and skills, and career goals. Individual traits which are important to the choice of research question include time management skills, ability to concentrate on a task and not be easily distracted, ability to think in a logical manner, patience, ability to write a structured flowing argument, and ability to be self-motivated. Other personal traits, such as ease with numerical or conceptual analyses, interpersonal communication skills and computer literacy, are also important considerations as these will make certain types of research, and hence research questions, more or less suitable for the individual.

The researching therapist's work experience and areas of expertise should also be analysed, as these will be used in conjunction with career goal information to decide whether to select a research question central to their current knowledge domain, or whether to extend that domain by selecting a question peripheral to their current knowledge.

The researching therapist's knowledge and skills related to research need to be analysed. An honest appraisal of knowledge of different types of qualitative or quantitative research, different measurement tools and analysis systems will be helpful when selecting an appropriate question. As for work experience and expertise, participation in research can be used to build on knowledge and skills or develop new areas. Building on an existing strong knowledge base will have the advantage of requiring less initial learning and a better understanding of the caveats associated with an area; the disadvantages will be a propensity to narrow vision and acceptance of assumptions which may be inappropriate.

Performing research takes considerable time and effort. It is therefore useful to have a clear indication of how involvement in a research project will further one's career and personal goals. This will help maintain motivation during the almost inevitable periods of difficulty. A clear view of career goals, including timeframes, will also be useful in the selection of a research question which will suit the career path chosen.

EXTENT AND NATURE OF THE LITERATURE BASE

An understanding of the literature knowledge base is a crucial preliminary step to choosing any research question. A researching therapist should already be familiar with the literature in their current area of work. However, if research is envisaged in other areas, then a review of the literature in those areas is important to assess the state of knowledge.

Research is easiest in areas where there is a strong existing literature base. Besides information about the topic, the literature may also provide theoretical models to assist a new researcher in conceptualizing the problems. A theoretical model is a way of organizing the knowledge into simple principles and relationships. A theory should provide a new researcher with an improved understanding of the area and ensure that important aspects are not missed.

Some qualitative methods require that the literature review be postponed until analysis of the data is completed. This is to ensure that the meaning of the data is derived from the data, and not forced on to the data by preconceptions.

The literature will also supply descriptions of study designs and methods used for the topic. One of the most useful aspects of the literature is being able to determine how effective various designs and methods have been. Even when the chosen research method excludes a review of literature on the research question, a review of research using similar research methods is advisable, as this will provide an insight into the practicalities of the methods as well as their philosophical underpinning. For example, if it was thought that grounded theory would be a useful method for a particular question, the researching therapist should review work on symbolic interactionism by Blumer (1969) and Glaser and Strauss (1967).

A reasonable view of the research in an area can usually be developed by reviewing journal articles published in the last 5 years; reviewing conference proceedings from the last 5 years (these usually describe more current research than journal articles, owing to the lengthy publication delays for many quality journals); and talking to experts in the field about work in progress.

 Key Points 3.1

Know one's own capacity

Learn from the documented experience of others

Know the available resources

NATURE AND AVAILABILITY OF OTHER RESOURCES

Other resources which need to be analysed include subjects, experts, equipment and related facilities, time, and funding possibilities.

Subjects/participants

Subjects is the term most commonly used in quantitative research, whereas participant is favoured by researchers doing qualitative research. Both terms are therefore used in this book.

Although many of the research topics of interest to therapists involve subjects, not all topics require live human participants. For example, research on the physiological effects of various treatment options frequently involves animals. Similarly, considerable background research of use to therapists has been performed on cadaveric tissue. However, research involving live humans is very popular with therapists owing to its perceived clinical relevance and significance. It has the advantages of being easily related to humans, does not require assumptions of generalizability from animal models, and may appear more relevant than cadaveric research.

However, the use of humans in research also brings possible problems. Research into the effectiveness of therapeutic interventions for a particular disorder relies on access to a willing subject population of an adequate size. Informal discussions with potential subjects may indicate their willingness to be involved. It should also be remembered that in many countries parental or guardian consent must be sought for participation by people under 18 years of age (see Chapter 7).

Randomized controlled trials need a definable degree of consistency in the subject groups. Thus disorders which are difficult to diagnose or categorize make the internal validity of controlled trials less secure. Such research may also be difficult owing to limited subject numbers. One approach sometimes taken to gain adequate numbers of subjects with rarer disorders is to collect data from a number of centres – termed a 'multicentre trial'. This is clearly important to identify early, as it will have considerable consequences for the viability of a research topic and on the detail of planning needed to ensure consistency across centres.

Knowing the types of subjects likely to be available, and the numbers of those potential participants, is important in determining an appropriate research topic.

Experts

Research is often complex, and many of the research topics of interest to therapists involve complex knowledge domains. Thus most researching therapists will need and use expert assistance at various stages of their research. Evaluating the types of expertise available is an important preliminary step to identifying a research topic.

All the knowledge and skill required for a particular study may be held by one expert or, more likely, a number of experts will be needed as resources for a particular study. The types of experts commonly used by therapists performing research can be grouped into several areas of knowledge and skill: research project management, research design and analysis, research methods, and clinical. Research project management expertise includes the knowledge and skills of project scheduling and time management, liaising with organizations and individuals participating in the study, subject recruitment through advertising and media interviews, and budget management.

Expertise in research design and analysis includes choosing a design suitable to the research question and available resources, determining sample size, proficiency with specific statistical or qualitative data management software, and data quality assurance and reduction.

Expertise in research methods relates to the specific methods and equipment likely to be used. For example, if focus groups form a major part of the intended study then the researching therapist needs access to someone with expertise in conducting focus groups. Similarly, if electromyography is to be used, then expertise with this method will be of great benefit. Finally, clinical expertise includes knowledge and skills covering the anatomical and physiological background, the pathology and the management of any disorders to be examined in the study.

In the evaluation of expert resources the researching therapist needs to locate individuals with the appropriate expertise and also to determine whether those individuals will be available when required, and whether they are willing to help.

Evaluation of whether an individual has the required expertise can be assisted by reviewing any related publications, attending talks by the individual, discussing issues of which the researching therapist has good knowledge, and through discussion with people who have attempted to use that individual as an expert resource.

Instruments and equipment

Although not all research topics are amenable to the use of equipment, the number of equipment items used by researching therapists (and their complexity) is increasing. Evaluation of the equipment available is important in determining suitable research topics.

The increasing pressure for quantified outcome measures for evaluating therapeutic inventions has resulted in a wide range of equipment being available to therapists. This extends from structured interview schedules to questionnaires; from simple mechanical devices such as a two-armed goniometer to complex electronic devices connected to computers. However, therapists should not be overawed by technology and should use equipment only when appropriate.

Some dependent variables require specific measuring equipment. Such requirements, and the availability of the necessary equipment, should be identified prior to selecting a research question.

Facilities

Facilities likely to be required for a research project include: room(s) of suitable size and features; transport for researcher and/or participants; library access; office space for organization and management of the project; telecommunications; photocopier, printer and computer.

Time

The time available and the expected date of project completion are important to identify early.

The types of research possible will vary depending on whether the therapist has taken a year out of clinical practice to complete a research project; is conducting the research as part of their employment and is happy to continue collecting data for 10 years; or is a student with programme time constraints.

The amount of time per week available for the research project should also be identified. The variability of time which can be committed to the research should be noted. For example, a therapist may be able to devote 6 hours a week to research for most of the year, but be willing and able to commit 20 hours a week for a number of weeks (perhaps for data collection) and may not be available at all for some other weeks (perhaps due to family commitments, holidays or exams). A clear concept of the time available will assist in choosing a suitable research topic.

Funding

Some research requires very little funding. For example, the costs of a qualitative evaluation of a single therapist–client interaction using videography may be small enough to be covered by the therapist or their employer/academic institution. If the study involves multiple interviews requiring transcription and analysis using computer software, the cost may be too great to be met by an individual. Similarly, studies requiring considerable printing and postage, purchase of research assistance or expertise, expensive diagnostic or treatment methods, or instrumentation, are likely to require separate funding. At the stage of choosing a research question which involves evaluating the therapist's current situation, all that is required is to ascertain the magnitude of likely funding required and whether such an amount is potentially available.

To determine whether funding for a particular project is likely, funding sources should be identified. By investigating the annual reports of these sources it should be possible to determine whether the common amount of funding is adequate, and whether the selected research topic is of interest to the organization. Chapter 8 provides more guidelines on applying for research funding.

EXAMPLE OF RESOURCE EVALUATION

The brief description which follows provides an illustration of the resource evaluation for a fictitious therapist (Therapist X).

Therapist X has good time management and communication skills. X has over 5 years' experience with clients who have had a cerebral vascular accident, and would like to understand what therapy means to them. X has no research background in qualitative methods but is very keen to develop some skills in that area. X's career and personal goals are to remain a clinician, but to gain increased work satisfaction by understanding the clients better.

X knows that there is considerable literature on therapy outcomes for this client group, and that although there is little qualitative research reported specific to this topic, there is sufficient to inform X of conceptual and methods issues.

X has access to around 50 suitable clients each year, and has collaborated on several small projects with a local academic who has considerable experience in heuristic and phenomenological methods. Working in a clinic, X has access to office space and equipment. X's personal commitments enable part-time study in addition to clinical work. The evaluation of quality of life outcomes is becoming increasingly important to the health insurance organization which finances X's clinic, and the organization has offered to fund research in this area.

Hazard 3.1

Failure to be honest in the appraisal of one's abilities and limitations is a common failure in evaluating research resources

This chapter has outlined many of the details a therapist needs to consider prior to selecting a research question. The following chapter describes the process of developing a research question once an appropriate question has been selected.

REFERENCES

Blumer H 1969 Symbolic interaction. Prentice-Hall, Englewood Cliffs, NJ
Glaser B, Strauss A 1967 The discovery of grounded theory. Aldine, Chicago

4 Developing a research question

Once a potentially researchable question has been chosen, it needs to be developed and refined. New researchers tend to start with a diffuse, global problem that is too complex or broad and is unlikely to be resolved through one investigation. The problem must therefore be reduced to a single answerable question: it may be necessary to split a general problem into a series of discrete research questions which can be investigated separately.

The process of developing and refining a research question establishes the limits or boundaries by narrowing the selected problem and by defining the scope of the investigation. Considerable time and thought are required to develop a research question, and it is recommended that the researching therapist discusses the issues highlighted in this chapter with colleagues and supervisors.

The development of the research question includes: determining what type of research is most appropriate to answer the question posed; refining the question by defining terms; listing assumptions and limitations; and refining the general research question into specific objectives and guiding questions, and possibly hypotheses, for the intended study.

IDENTIFYING THE TYPE OF RESEARCH

An important aspect of developing a research question is to identify the type of question. Some require little or no analysis, whereas others require considerable abstraction and analysis of data. Further, some research questions are more suited to quantitative methods, whereas others are more suited to qualitative approaches.

Descriptive questions tend to appear fairly simple and ask 'What is A like?'. Descriptive designs may include case studies, programme evaluations, historical surveys, action research and ethnographic or phenomenological case studies. Examples of both qualitative and quantitative descriptive research questions include:

- *What is the trunk strength of elite hockey players?*
- *What is the treatment and rehabilitation experience of people who have had severe burns?*
- *How do Western Australian adolescents perform on the Screening for Auditory Processing Disorders test?*
- *What is the compliance of clients with amputations with prosthesis care instructions?*

Research questions which require more analysis ask things like: 'Is A related to B?', 'Does A cause C?'. More analytical designs may include grounded theory, correlation studies, quasi-experimental designs, small *n*/time series analyses, randomized control trials, naturalistic interpretive enquiries and repeated measures factorial studies. Examples include:

- *Is trunk strength in a group of elite hockey players who have performed 6 weeks of specific trunk exercises different from that of a group of elite hockey players who have performed no specific trunk exercises (i.e. does performing specific trunk exercises increase trunk strength in elite hockey players)?*
- *Is the client perception of client–therapist communication different in interactions with a group of therapists trained in communication skills than in interactions with a group of therapists with no training in communication skills (i.e. does training in communication skills improve the client's perception of client–therapist communication)?*
- *Is the auditory processing ability of adolescents with learning disorders better in those who have completed the metalinguistic training programme than in those who have not completed such a programme (i.e. does metalinguistic training*

benefit auditory processing ability in learning-disabled adolescents)?
- *Is prosthesis life related to client attitudes to prosthesis care?*

As can be seen, the types of research questions tend to merge with each other and it is often difficult to categorize the question type clearly. (For example, 'What is A like?' could be asking about the conceptual model clients have – which may require high-level abstraction and analysis.) However, having an idea of the type of research question helps establish some of the boundaries for an intended study: for instance, it narrows the possibilities for appropriate study designs. It also provides a quick method for describing important aspects of the research question and so facilitates concise discussion with colleagues.

DEFINING TERMS

In research it is vital to be explicit and precise. Thus any terms to be used in the research question and in the subsequent research should be defined to avoid misinterpretation. This is particularly important when discussing key concepts, performance indicators and variables. Suitable definitions can be taken from quality sources such as peer-reviewed journals, respected books and dictionaries.

Defining a variable is often described as operationalizing a term, that is, defining exactly what the variable is by saying how one would actually go about measuring it. For example, one may be interested in whether a regular exercise programme reduces the pain suffered by patients with low back pain. The independent variable 'regular exercise programme' and the dependent variable 'pain' need further defining before the reader knows exactly what is meant. As mentioned, one of the aspects of defining a variable is to say how it will be measured. 'Regular exercise' would need to be defined in terms of the nature of the exercise (e.g. the types of movements performed, their speed, energy requirements, duration of exercise periods) and its frequency. 'Pain' could be measured by subjective ratings of magnitude, location and nature, by diaries of temporal patterns, by observable behaviours or even by physiological correlates such as galvanic skin response, static muscle activity and heart rate. Thus, although regular exercise and pain appear fairly small concepts, they are in fact quite broad and should be clarified in any research description.

In programme evaluation studies it may be important to define the objectives of the programme and the performance indicators used.

Another way of helping to define the terms used in a research project is to develop a model (or use a model which is already developed, with appropriate referencing). A model is a simplified representation of something more complex. For example, in researching the assessment of manual handling one could use a model like that of Straker (1994, p. 69) to help explain the factors that could affect permissible risk (Fig. 4.1). Models are very useful for illustrating relationships.

If it is not possible to adequately define a key concept or variable, or if there is no coherent model available, qualitative methods could be used to provide them. This requires changing the research question from something like 'Does A relate to B?' to 'What is A?'.

DECLARING ASSUMPTIONS, BIASES AND PERSPECTIVES

Stating the assumptions helps to document

where the therapist 'is coming from'. According to Bailey (1991, p. 77), 'Assumptions are underlying principles that the researcher believes or accepts but that are difficult to prove in any concrete way. They are frequently untested and untestable hypotheses, basic values, or views about the world'. For example, a report by Smith (1996) states in the opening paragraph that it 'is based on a qualitative, feminist sociological study' of therapy assistants.

Assumptions can also determine what approach is taken to a specific situation. For example, if the research question were *What is the outcome following an intensive inpatient exercise programme for patients with ankylosing spondylitis?*, various approaches could be taken to answer it. A health economist working on the assumption that the community must obtain value for the funds it has contributed to the programme may evaluate the costs of the programme and the expected savings based on estimates of improved productivity and reduced morbidity of participants. A social worker using the assumption that the most important aspect of intervention is the patient's perception of the outcome, may evaluate that outcome in terms of participants' perceived improvement in quality of life.

Whereas qualitative researchers are frequently explicit in their assumptions of perspectives, quantitative researchers tend unadvisedly to ignore their assumptions. Payton (1988) lists a number of assumptions of the scientific method. These include that science is objective; that the behaviour of the universe is consistent; that knowledge is only tentative; that every phenomenon results from a discoverable cause; and (contradicting the first assumption) that the society within which the scientist works will influence the research performed and the interpretation of the data. These are all assumptions about the research process in general.

There are also assumptions pertinent to each study. For example, it may be necessary to assume that subjects perform with the same honesty and effort on each occasion, and that the instruments perform reliably on each occasion. Noting the assumptions helps one to consider how a study could be improved, for example by

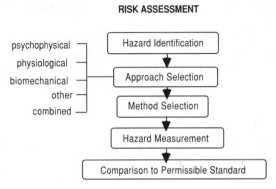

Figure 4.1 A manual handling risk assessment model (Straker, 1994)

taking steps to ensure that potentially motivating factors are equal on each occasion, and by calibrating equipment regularly.

Every study has assumptions. If all these are listed the researching therapist may wonder, *Why bother*? However, it is an important part in understanding the tentative nature of scientific knowledge. The assumptions which are specific to the chosen study, and which may influence the results, need to be documented so that they are available when the results are interpreted.

IDENTIFYING LIMITATIONS

Similarly, one should be aware of the limitations of the research and make the audience aware of these in any communication. Limitations could include shortcomings with the methods, such as lack of randomization or control, lack of standardized instruments or limitation of sample size. Limitations also include deficiencies in the theories and concepts applied in the study. For example, the theory may be very controversial, or not very detailed, or non-existent.

Key Point 4.1

Time spent in careful development of the research question will pay dividends in a better quality project and less time wasted performing the project.

GOING FROM GENERAL TO SPECIFIC

To understand the process of refining a question, it may be useful to consider a hierarchy going from general to specific. This hierarchy would start with the problem, question and aim at the more general levels, become more specific through objectives and end with either specific guiding questions or hypotheses.

The problem

At the most general level is the problem. This is a simple statement of what is.

Example 1 There is no information on how many speech therapists work in schools in Western Australia.

Example 2 The nature of older people's physical activity is not known.

Example 3 It is not known whether treatment A or treatment B is more effective for reducing swelling.

Example 4 Some patients respond better to treatment A than others and it is not known why.

The question

The question follows from the problem, converting the problem into something that can be answered.

Example 1 How many speech therapists work in schools in Western Australia?

Example 2 What is the experience of physical activity of a group of older people?

Example 3 Is treatment A or B more effective for reducing swelling?

Example 4 Why do some patients respond better to treatment A than other patients?

The aim

The aim, sometimes called the purpose, of the project is to solve the problem and answer the question.

The aim of this study is:

Example 1 to determine how many speech therapists work in schools.

Example 2 to explore the activities of and the importance of those activities to a group of older people.

Example 3 to determine which treatment, A or B, is more effective in reducing swelling.

Example 4 to determine why some patients respond better to treatment A than other patients.

Objectives

The objectives are more specific than the aim, and say what the researcher is going to do. There will usually be a number of specific objectives for each aim.

The specific objectives of this study are to:

Example 1

- collect information from all primary and secondary schools in Western Australia on the number of speech therapists who work in these schools
- compare the number of female and male speech therapists working in schools in Western Australia
- compare the number of speech therapists working in primary and secondary schools in Western Australia
- compare the number of speech therapists and their pattern of involvement with schools in Western Australia with the number of speech therapists and their pattern of involvement in schools in other Australian states.

Example 2

- observe the physical activities and relationships of people attending a senior citizen's activity centre at various times of the day
- explore the meaning of the activities in relation to the individuals attending the centre
- explore the perceptions of the individuals regarding their previous and current levels of activity.

Example 3

- collect data on the effectiveness of ultrasound and interferential therapy in reducing swelling following an acute ankle injury
- compare the effectiveness of the two treatments
- compare the findings of this study with other studies
- provide guidelines for choosing an appropriate electrotherapy treatment for reducing swelling following an acute ankle injury.

Example 4

- collect ratings of wellbeing before and after participation in exercise classes from a group of patients with depression and a group of patients with mania
- collect ratings of wellbeing from matched groups of patients with depression and mania not participating in exercise classes
- determine the effect of participation in an exercise class on the ratings of wellbeing by psychologically disturbed patients
- determine the effect of type of psychological disturbance, depression or mania, on ratings of wellbeing

- determine whether the type of psychological disturbance alters the effect of exercise class participation.

Specific guiding questions or hypotheses

Each objective should have a specific guiding question (G) and/or a hypothesis (H). Hypotheses operationalize objectives which are to be tested statistically, and so not all objectives will have hypotheses (see Chapter 5 for more details).

Example 1

G How many speech therapists, what is their gender and what are their tasks, in primary and secondary schools in Western Australia.

H There are proportionally more male than female speech therapists working in Western Australian schools.

H There are more speech therapists working in primary schools than secondary schools in Western Australia.

H/G There are proportionally fewer speech therapists working in schools in Western Australia than in Victoria or New South Wales. What are the apparent differences in tasks performed by speech therapists in schools in Western Australia compared with schools in Victoria and New South Wales?

Example 2

G What are the activities and relationships of people attending a senior citizens' centre?

G What is meaning of these activities to this particular group? What is the meaning of the relationships developed to this particular group?

G What is the past and present activity experience of the people attending a senior citizens' centre? What are their perceptions of this experience? What factors promote a feeling of wellbeing? What factors hinder a feeling of wellbeing?

Example 3

G What are the measures of ankle swelling before and after ultrasound and interferential therapy?

H There is a greater reduction in swelling of patients with acute ankle ligament tears, as measured by immersion, following pulsed ultrasound than following interferential therapy.

G   How do the results of this study compare with other studies?

G   What guidelines can be given on appropriate therapy for ankle swelling?

Example 4

G   What are the ratings of wellbeing before and after participation in an exercise class for patients with depression and mania?

G   What are the ratings of wellbeing of patients with depression and mania who do not participate in exercise classes?

H   The ratings of wellbeing are higher in a group of psychologically disturbed patients who have participated in an exercise class than in a matched group of patients who have watched a video of an exercise class.

H   The ratings of wellbeing are higher in patients with mania who have participated in an exercise class than in patients with depression who have participated in the same class.

H   There is an interaction between the type of psychological disturbance and participation in an exercise class, such that the ratings of wellbeing by patients with depression are increased more than the ratings by patients with mania.

Most types of research benefit from the clarity of direction provided by the early development of explicit objectives and guiding questions/ hypotheses. However, this is not possible or suitable for some research questions and approaches, as the aspects of importance only become apparent during data collection. For example, if the problem were that factors which influence compliance with therapy intervention in patients with muscular dystrophy was not known, the aim would be to identify those factors. However, it may not be possible to be specific about the guiding questions until the actual factors, such as fear of death, boredom with therapy, loss of valuable time, are identified.

Hazard 4.1

Drifting away from the research question with the guiding questions/hypotheses so that the research question will not be adequately answered

Trying to answer too large a question/too many guiding questions/hypotheses

Ignoring research resources when developing the guiding questions/hypotheses

Thinking qualitative or quantitative research is better/worse

Not recognizing biases and limitations

This chapter has described how to develop a selected research question. At this stage in the research process the researching therapist should be able to discuss concisely their ideas with colleagues, including the type of study envisaged, the limitations and assumptions and the specific guiding questions and hypotheses to be addressed. Once the question has been developed to this extent a formal proposal should be developed. Chapter 5 provides guidelines for the writing of a research proposal.

REFERENCES

Bailey D M 1991 Research for the health professional: a practical guide. F A Davis, Philadelphia

Payton O D 1988 Research: the validation of clinical practice, 2nd edn. F A Davis, Philadelphia

Smith S 1996 Ethnographic inquiry in physiotherapy research: 1 Illuminating the working culture of the physiotherapy assistant. Physiotherapy 82(6): 342–352

Straker L M 1994 Risk assessment in combination manual handling tasks. Unpublished doctoral thesis, University of Sydney, Sydney

5 Writing a research proposal

A research proposal is a written plan which includes a statement of the problem to be investigated and its importance, the research question(s)/hypotheses to be answered/tested, and the research protocol. The proposal has a number of important functions: it illustrates to the reviewers the researcher's critical thinking on the research topic and synthesis of the supporting literature; demonstrates that the research is based on sound theoretical rationale; shows that the methods proposed are appropriate for answering the question; serves as the working document enabling communication between members of a research team; and during the data collecting phase of the study, the protocol provides the guide to the processes involved.

This chapter serves as a general guide to the structure and content of a proposal. Proposals are often written as part of the assessment for an undergraduate or postgraduate research unit, for higher degree studies, or form part of a grant application. In such cases the length and format of the proposal, including the headings for the individual sections, are usually specified.

STRUCTURE OF A PROPOSAL

A proposal is typically divided into a number of sections; the principal sections provide an introduction to the research topic (Introduction), discuss the relevant background literature (Literature Review) and describe the methods (Methods). To improve clarity, the Literature Review and the Methods are usually subdivided into relevant areas, often with numbered headings (Fig. 5.1). Proposals should also include a section on the resources required and an estimate of costs. Appendices may be attached to the proposal (see p. 36 for examples of information which may be placed in an appendix). Proposals for grant applications and for other research purposes may require an Abstract and a separate section which discusses the significance of the research (this is otherwise addressed in the Introduction). When applying for a grant, the proposal must contain a detailed budget (see Chapter 8 p. 57–58).

Writing style and verb tense

The proposal must be written in a scientific style (see Chapter 14). It describes a study that will take place in the future; the researcher's thinking about the problem is taking place now and hence is written in the *present tense*. The Literature Review covers work that has been published, and so the *past tense* is used. The Methods section deals with what is going to be done, and is written in the *future tense*.

THE PROPOSAL

The remainder of this chapter is divided into sections corresponding to the sections of a proposal, and there is reference throughout to other chapters which contain information to assist with the development and writing of the proposal.

Title

The title provides the first impression to the reader. It must be concise and clearly reflect the nature of the study, i.e. the title must have some relationship to the hypotheses or guiding questions. For example, the title *Cystic Fibrosis* conveys very little to the reader and does not suggest that any research on the topic will be undertaken. Expanding the title to *Effects of Exercise Training on Airway Clearance in Adolescent Subjects with Cystic Fibrosis* gives the reader a good deal of information. It suggests that research will be undertaken and that there is both an independent variable

(exercise training) and a dependent variable (airway clearance). The title also specifies the age of the subject population. An effective title should include all essential keywords that fully and accurately convey the study content. Only the necessary words should be used and all redundant words removed (e.g. *A study of*). Finally, the order of the words should be such that they accurately reflect the intended meaning.

Preliminary pages

The preliminary pages (those pages prior to the Introduction) may include a list of abbreviations used in the proposal and definitions of technical terms. A table of contents is only necessary for a long proposal.

Introduction

The Introduction should tell the reader what the problem is and why it is worthy of study. The statement of the research question is the most important statement in the Introduction. The section usually concludes by stating the main aim(s) of the study.

In order to awaken the reader's interest, the Introduction needs to be direct and to the point. Therefore, it should be as short as possible (often one or two pages) while still achieving clarity and being informative. The aim is to excite the reader so that they feel compelled to read further and discover more about the intended study.

The Introduction should begin with a clear statement of the problem in terms which can be easily understood by the reader. At this stage the reader will generally be unfamiliar with the technicalities of the study, including technical terminology; these will be introduced later. The problem statement must provide the rationale for the research question, thereby providing a logical progression from identification of the problem through to the research question (see Chapter 4).

The next section of the Introduction should begin by clarifying why the topic is significant, together with the relevant support. In the case of a clinical study the significance may be expressed in terms of the number of people with the prob-

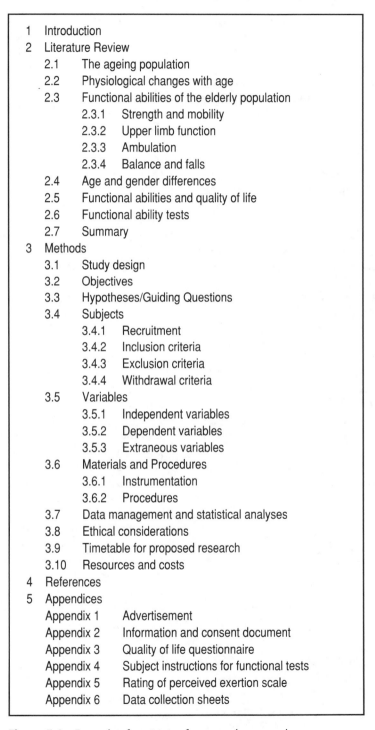

1   Introduction
2   Literature Review
    2.1   The ageing population
    2.2   Physiological changes with age
    2.3   Functional abilities of the elderly population
        2.3.1   Strength and mobility
        2.3.2   Upper limb function
        2.3.3   Ambulation
        2.3.4   Balance and falls
    2.4   Age and gender differences
    2.5   Functional abilities and quality of life
    2.6   Functional ability tests
    2.7   Summary
3   Methods
    3.1   Study design
    3.2   Objectives
    3.3   Hypotheses/Guiding Questions
    3.4   Subjects
        3.4.1   Recruitment
        3.4.2   Inclusion criteria
        3.4.3   Exclusion criteria
        3.4.4   Withdrawal criteria
    3.5   Variables
        3.5.1   Independent variables
        3.5.2   Dependent variables
        3.5.3   Extraneous variables
    3.6   Materials and Procedures
        3.6.1   Instrumentation
        3.6.2   Procedures
    3.7   Data management and statistical analyses
    3.8   Ethical considerations
    3.9   Timetable for proposed research
    3.10   Resources and costs
4   References
5   Appendices
    Appendix 1   Advertisement
    Appendix 2   Information and consent document
    Appendix 3   Quality of life questionnaire
    Appendix 4   Subject instructions for functional tests
    Appendix 5   Rating of perceived exertion scale
    Appendix 6   Data collection sheets

Figure 5.1   Example of contents of a research proposal

lem, the impact of the problem on the community (e.g. patient days in hospital, employment days lost) and the cost to those with the problem (e.g. impaired quality of life).

The final paragraph(s) is used to state the research question(s) and the main aim(s) of the study.

Literature Review

A literature Review combines the summaries and critical analyses of a number of articles grouped to cover the important topics/issues addressed in the review. For each topic a summary of the main findings from the literature should be presented, followed by an evaluation of the quality of support for those findings (identified in the critique of each article). The value of the reported work must be judged and commented upon. In particular, conflicting data must be discussed. A mere descriptive account of the literature does not constitute a literature review. Where data are discussed, the International System of Units (SI) should be used throughout; consequently, data from some published studies may need to be converted. Statements that are currently true are written in the *present tense*. This is used when stating the question. The *past tense* is used when referring to findings, or what researchers have thought or done in the past. The contents of a Literature Review are outlined in Key Points 5.1.

Key Points 5.1

Literature Review

Contents   Overview of structure and content

Summary and critique of comparable research which has been published relating to the problem or components of the problem

Critique of the methods available for answering the research question

A final one-paragraph summary of the literature, which is then related to the proposed area of study

It is helpful to both the writer and the reader if the review begins with an opening paragraph which states its boundaries and gives an overview of its structure. For example, a literature review of the use of early ambulation in the management of patients undergoing cardiac surgery could begin with the statement: *This review covers the use of early ambulation in the management of patients undergoing cardiac surgery. The review is confined to a discussion of the literature from 1980 to the present. The following related physiotherapeutic techniques are outside the scope of this review: positioning, upper limb exercises and lower limb exercises during bed rest. The review concludes with an examination of the methods available for measuring the efficacy of ambulation as a treatment strategy.*

The extent of the Literature Review will depend on the nature of the study. Both the most recent literature and significant older references should be included. The definition of what constitutes recent literature will vary depending on the topic.

Some qualitative methodologies (e.g. phenomenology) may require that literature relating to the area of study not be reviewed until after analysis has been completed. In the proposal, however, it is necessary to demonstrate that the researcher has the knowledge and understanding to carry out the research. The literature which is reviewed will need to reflect an understanding of these principles and be substantiated by critical analysis of literature on viable methods. The Literature Review must include the key references necessary for evaluating the problem. It is important to keep in mind that the literature discussed must provide the relevant information to support the research question, the rationale for the methods chosen and the justification for the study. The number of references will vary depending on the topic of the research and, in some instances, a maximum number may be set in the guidelines for the proposal. Even when a limit is not provided, it is essential to restrict the number of references by ensuring that only the key ones are used. The references selected should be the most important, the most valid, those which are most easily available and, where appropriate, the most recent (see Chapter 14 p. 105–106).

The Literature Review should conclude with a summary of the knowledge that is well supported and an indication of what is unknown or what requires further support in relation to the proposed area of study.

Methods

This is invariably the longest section of the proposal. It describes in full the subject / participant sample, exact details of what will be done, when, how and by whom. The level of detail must be sufficient so that the soundness of the study and its feasibility can be determined by those reviewing the proposal. The following sections provide more information relating to aspects of the Methods which should be included in the proposal. A summary of the information is provided in Key Points 5.2.

Outline of study design

The type of study design should be stated; for example:

- *An experimental design will be used with subjects randomly allocated to either treatment or control groups.*
- *A prospective, longitudinal study design will be used.*
- *A single subject experimental design (ABAB) will be used.*
- *An ethnographic approach will be used.*

The statement of the research design should make clear whether it incorporates independent or repeated factors.

Objectives

These should be presented in chronological order, order of importance or ordered to be consistent with the hypotheses or guiding questions (examples of objectives can be found in Chapter 4 p. 24–25).

Hypotheses/guiding questions

Hypotheses are generated for experimental,

Key Points 5.2

Methods

Contents	The order of presentation of the information may vary depending on the study and on the type of research approach
Outline of study design	Description of overall study design that will be used to test the research hypothesis(es) or answer the guiding question(s)
Objectives	Complete list of study objectives
Hypothesis(es) or guiding questions	Statement of the hypothesis(es) or guiding questions that will be answered regarding the sample
Subjects/ Participants	Method of recruitment, estimate of number and justification of sample size (including a power analysis when required)
	Inclusion, exclusion and withdrawal criteria
	Method of allocation to study groups
Variables	Operational definitions of independent and dependent variables
	List of extraneous variables and how they will be controlled (when possible)
Materials	Equipment, instruments or measurement tools
	Calibration, validity and reliability
Procedures for data collection	Environment (research venue) where the study will take place
	Presentation in chronological order of what will be done, when, how and by whom
	Methods to ensure scientific rigour of data (e.g. video recording, field notes, memos)
Pilot studies	Purpose of any pilot studies, subjects/participants, procedures
	Outcome/results, modifications to methods for main study

Key Points 5.2 (*cont'd*)

Data management and analyses	Method of storage of data and access
	Proposed method for data examination including methods of dealing with outlying data and reducing data to format required for any statistical analyses
	Description of computer programs (including version or release number) which will be used for data management and analysis (e.g. The Ethnograph, Hyperqual, SPSS, SAS) or description of cut and paste methods. Description of coding, content analysis and constant comparison, with appropriate references to support method
	Specific tests, including names of tests and whether one-tailed or two-tailed, critical α probability (*P*) value taken to represent statistical significance, appropriate references to support choice of less commonly used tests (e.g. post hoc comparisons)
Ethical considerations	Clear statement of the ethical aspects of the study (a copy of the documentation of informed consent should be attached as an appendix to the proposal)
Timetable for proposed research	Dates for each stage of the research process, including timelines for communication of findings in verbal/poster and written formats
Identification of resources and budget	List of all resources required for the project, including costs where appropriate

quasi-experimental and correlational studies. It is recommended, where possible, that hypotheses are generated for reliability studies.

The research hypothesis (also known as the alternative hypothesis or the experimental hypothesis) is stated within the proposal and declares the researcher's true expectations of the results. Current scientific practice is to design a study to reject the null hypothesis (H_0), with the only plausible alternative being the research hypothesis. The data obtained in the study are analysed by testing H_0, which expresses no relationship or no difference between the variables.

The phrasing of the research hypothesis may be such that the direction of a difference is predicted (directional hypothesis). Alternatively, the research hypothesis may merely state that there will be a difference (non-directional hypothesis). The symbol used to represent the research hypothesis is usually H_A or, if several hypotheses have been generated, they are numbered consecutively (H_1, H_2, H_3, etc.).

On occasions the relationship between variables may be expressed in the form of a complex hypothesis (i.e. a hypothesis which contains more than one independent variable (IV) and one dependent variable (DV)). Such a hypothesis provides a succinct means of expressing the expected outcome of a study. The following are examples of different types of hypotheses.

Directional
Subjects who smoke cigarettes have a greater chance of developing ischaemic heart disease than subjects who do not smoke cigarettes.

Non-directional
There is a difference in anxiety levels, as measured using a standardized questionnaire, between patients who receive preoperative education and those who do not.

Complex
Low-intensity static exercise involving the upper limbs is associated with a significant increase in heart rate, as measured using a cardiac monitor, and arterial blood pressure, as measured using an automated blood pressure monitor.

Hypothesis for a reliability study
Experienced therapists are more reliable than new graduates in their ability to predict successful outcome of patients following discharge from hospital.

Qualitative studies, for example questionnaire surveys or ethnography using extensive interviews and focus group data, may not have hypotheses but instead have guiding questions, which make clear what the researcher is trying to find out and set the boundaries of the study. The following guiding questions might be developed for a study designed to gather information, using a questionnaire survey, from general practitioners (GPs) regarding their perceptions of the value of occupational therapists, physiotherapists and speech therapists as members of the primary health-care team.

1. *What are the perceptions of GPs regarding the role of occupational therapists, physiotherapists and speech therapists within the primary health-care team?*
2. *What is the extent of referral of patients, by GPs, to occupational therapists, physiotherapists and speech therapists?*
3. *What proportion of GPs consider that it would be of benefit to have occupational therapists, physiotherapists and speech therapists attached to their practices?*

Subjects/participants

The term 'subject' is generally used in experimental, quasi-experimental and correlational studies when referring to the participants (e.g. patients, therapists, healthy individuals) in a study. In qualitative research all individuals, including the researcher, are considered to be participants. For brevity, the term 'subject' has been used in the following discussion.

The details of the subjects must include how many, from where they will be recruited and the method of recruitment (e.g. in response to advertisements placed on noticeboards in the university). If subjects are to be allocated to study groups the method of allocation is required. Subject characteristics such as gender, age, height, weight, diagnosis, level of disability or duration of hospitalization must be defined when relevant to the study.

The following provides an example of the inclusion, exclusion and withdrawal criteria for a study investigating the effect of body posture on wheelchair stability.

Inclusion criteria
The sample will consist of 30 non-disabled subjects *aged between 18 and 50 years. An equal number of males and females will be studied. Only subjects who give written, informed consent will be studied.*

Exclusion criteria
Subjects will be excluded from the study if any of the following criteria apply:

i) *Inability to understand written or spoken English*
ii) *Presence or recent history (previous 6 months) of musculoskeletal problems affecting the cervical, thoracic or lumbar spine, shoulder girdle or upper limbs*
iii) *Body mass index of less than 18 or more than 28*
iv) *Pregnancy.*

Withdrawal criteria
Subjects will be withdrawn from the study in the event of any of the following:

i) *Withdrawal of consent*
ii) *Development of musculoskeletal abnormalities during the period of the study.*

Hazard 5.1

A common error is the confusion over the terms exclusion and withdrawal. A subject who is withdrawn satisfied the inclusion criteria but then for some reason had to be withdrawn, often because the continued presence of the subject in the study is thought likely to interfere with the quality of the data

Variables

The variables of interest, i.e. the IV, DV and extraneous variables (also called intervening variables), in the study must be stated in operational terms, for example specifying the procedures and the equipment used when making a measurement. The means of controlling (when possible) potential extraneous variables should also be stated. The use of operational definitions for variables should ensure that another suitably qualified person will have enough information to replicate the study. The following are examples of the level of detail required when describing variables.

Description of variables The following might

be a treatment regimen (IV) used in a study of physiotherapy for patients with osteoarthritis of the knee joint.

Subjects allocated to the intervention group will receive two supervised sessions of physiotherapy each week. Sessions will last for 15 minutes each. Subjects will perform three sets of 10 repetitions of the following exercises: inner range quadriceps over an 18 cm wooden block, straight leg raises to a height of 18 cm and isometric quadriceps contractions. Subjects will be instructed to perform the exercises twice per day during the 4-week study period and will be provided with a diary in which to record exercise sessions.

In the above study quadriceps strength (DV) is to be measured at weekly intervals. The operational definition of the DV might be as follows:

Quadriceps strength will be measured using a KinCom 500H computer-controlled isokinetic dynamometer (Chattecx Group, Hixson, Tennessee, USA). Subjects will be tested sitting with the lever arm strapped, using a cushioned shin pad, to the subject's leg just above the level of the malleoli. With the knee joint at 90° of flexion, the dynamometer will be aligned to the joint axis of rotation. Subjects will be given a period of familiarization with the procedures during which at least three trials will be performed, before measurements are made. Concentric torque will be measured from 90° of knee flexion to the maximum extension a subject can reach at a speed of 90° per second. Three maximum voluntary contractions will be separated by 20-second recovery periods.

The extraneous variables likely to influence the outcome of this quadriceps strength study are medication taken by subjects and the amount of physical activity. The proposal must include the methods by which such variables will be controlled. For example:

Subjects will be instructed to keep constant the dose and frequency of any medication. They will be told to continue with their normal level of physical activity (activities of daily living, walking) and not to take up any new activities, such as sports, during the study period. An activity log will be provided for subjects to record their daily physical activity.

Materials and procedures

The exact model, brand name and manufacturer

Hazard 5.2

A common error is the incorrect use of the word 'dependant' when referring to the dependent variable

The term 'regime' is often used incorrectly. When referring to a prescribed course of exercises or a treatment programme, the correct term is 'regimen'. A 'regime' is a governmental or social system

(name, city and country of address) must be given in the description of all commercially available equipment. The method of calibration of all equipment should be given (full details can be included in an appendix if a lengthy process has to be followed). This section of the proposal gives details of the procedures for data collection; the procedures for recruiting subjects are included in the 'Subjects/Participants' section. If any of the procedures are very lengthy, then a brief description can be provided within the text and the full description given in an appendix. Alternatively, reference can be made to a published paper, attached as an appendix, which presents all the details in full.

Hazard 5.3

'Data' is a plural term: 'datum' is the singular term. *Data was analysed* is a common error encountered; the correct form is: *Data were analysed*

Pilot studies

These are invariably vital to a successful study and are undertaken for a variety of reasons (e.g. reliability or validity testing of instrumentation; tester reliability; to identify ambiguous questions in a questionnaire; to estimate the time needed to complete data collection; to reveal unforeseen limitations in study design and allow modifications; trial procedures for data collection; to test the data collection forms; to identify and control or eliminate extraneous variables; to provide sample data for pilot data management and analysis procedures). The proposal should include an outline of any pilot studies which will be carried out prior to the main study. If pilot studies have already been completed at the time of writing the proposal, then the outcomes from these should be included together with information as to how the main study has been developed in the light of the findings.

Hazard 5.4

A common error encountered by reviewers of proposals is failure to provide sufficient information in the Methods. The point to constantly bear in mind when writing the Methods is that the reader should have all the information necessary to carry out the study. The reviewers must have enough detail so that the appropriateness of the study and its feasibility can be judged

Ethical considerations

A statement of the ethical considerations of the study should be included and a copy of the information consent document included in an appendix (see Chapter 7).

Timetable for proposed research

The timetable should list the major tasks and the time required to complete them. The estimates of time may be given as specific dates or in weeks or months, depending on the requirements listed in the guidelines for the proposal. The timetable should also include the time required for preparing communications of the findings (e.g. conference presentation, journal manuscript, research report or thesis). A common failure is to leave the writing up until all the data have been collected and analysed. Once pilot studies have been completed, the written description should not be left until completion of the main study. Delay with the preparation of written reports may well cause problems in meeting submission dates.

The following list provides examples of the types of tasks to be considered in the timetable; additional information to assist with project timings can be found in Chapter 11.

- Familiarization with equipment and testing procedures
- Familiarization with data management systems and software for data analysis
- Pilot study(ies) and refinement of procedures
- Preparation of advertisements and recruitment of subjects
- Main study data collection
- Write up Methods
- Data reduction and data analyses
- Write Results, including preparation of tables and figures
- Write Discussion
- Write Conclusions/Summary
- Revise Introduction/Literature Review
- Complete References and Acknowledgements
- Write Abstract
- Prepare for conference presentations
- Prepare journal manuscript.

Identification of resources and budget

An evaluation of the research resources will have been conducted prior to finalizing the research question (see Chapter 3). All proposals should include details of all the resources required and an estimate of the expenses which will be incurred. This information is essential so that the reviewers can assess the feasibility of the project. Resources may include subjects, experts, equipment and related facilities, time and funding possibilities, and the list should identify when and for how long each is required. Financial costs may include such items as photocopying, postage, telephone calls, reimbursement of travel expenses for subjects, computer disks, electrodes, costs associated with the development of a new instrument, and the cost of any procedures (e.g. scans, X-rays) required solely for the purposes of the study. For more details on research resources and the research budget, see Chapters 3 and 8.

References

These should start on a new page and the list should contain only those references which are cited within the proposal. A recognized system should be used for referencing: this may be specified in the guidelines for the proposal (see Chapter 14 p. 106).

Appendices

Appendices should be numbered in sequence as mentioned in the text, and each should start on a new page. Depending on the institutional guidelines for the proposal, any or all of the following may be included in an appendix:

- Copies of any advertisements and letters relating to subject recruitment
- Details of calibration procedures
- Full description of any lengthy procedures
- Copies of any original scales or questionnaires
- Verbatim instructions to subjects
- Copies of data collection forms
- Informed consent document
- Evidence of ethics approval (if already obtained).

The planning and writing of a proposal is invariably a very time-consuming activity. The writer should expect to have to revise and edit part or all of the proposal many times. During all stages of the development of the proposal, it is vital to obtain review from others (see Chapter 14 p. 108).

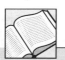

Further Reading

Bailey D M 1991 Research for the health professionals: a practical guide. F A Davis, Philadelphia

Bork C E 1993 Research in physical therapy. Lippincott, Philadelphia

Cohen J 1988 Statistical power for the behavioural sciences, 2nd edn. Erlbaum, Hillsdale, NJ

Currie D P 1990 Elements in research in physical therapy, 3rd edn. Williams & Wilkins, Baltimore

Denzin N Z, Lincoln Y S (eds) 1994 Handbook of qualitative research. Sage Publications, Thousand Oaks

DePoy E, Gitlin L N 1994 Introduction to research. Mosby, St. Louis

Further Reading (*cont'd*)

Domholdt E 1993 Physical therapy research: principles and applications. W B Saunders, Philadelphia

Fisher L D, Van Belle G 1993 Biostatistics: a methodology for the health sciences. John Wiley, New York

Glaser B G (ed) 1993 Examples of grounded theory: a reader. Sociology Press, Mill Valley

Hicks C M 1995 Research for physiotherapists: project design and analysis, 2nd edn. Churchill Livingstone, Edinburgh

Hulley S B, Cummings S (eds) 1988 Designing clinical research: an epidemiological approach. Williams & Wilkins, Baltimore

Laposata M 1992 SI unit conversion guide NEJM Books, Boston

Lewith G T, Aldridge D (eds) 1993 Clinical research methodology for complementary therapies. Hodder & Stoughton, London

Payton O D 1994 Research: the validation of clinical practice, 3rd edn. F A Davis, Philadelphia

Polgar S, Thomas S A 1995 Introduction to research in the health sciences, 3rd edn. Churchill Livingstone, Melbourne

Portney L G, Watkins M P 1993 Foundations of clinical research: applications to practice. Appleton and Lange, Connecticut, pp. 100–102

Rudestam K E, Newton R R 1992 Surviving your dissertation. Sage Publications, London

6 Presenting the research proposal

The development of the research proposal is an extremely focused activity in which material and ideas from a number of sources are collected and integrated and a new direction for research is formulated and outlined. During this process only those directly involved in the project (i.e. the researching therapist(s) and supervisor(s)) will have a clear understanding of it. Consequently it may be desirable – or indeed part of the requirements of a course of study – to present the proposal to members of the professional and research community so that the work may be scrutinized prior to implementing the study. This chapter emphasizes the importance of this process and outlines the contents and structure of the presentation. Further details regarding presentations may be found in Chapter 19.

PURPOSE

The presentation of the proposal is an important stage in the research process as it signals the transition between preparation and action. The timing of the presentation is important, and the researcher should plan to make the presentation well in advance of submitting the written proposal. Adequate lead time must be allowed so that any suggested modifications can be incorporated into the final proposal. These suggestions generally strengthen the proposal and may help to prevent delays in gaining approval for the project. In some institutions a written summary of the proposal is made available to potential members of the audience in advance of the presentation. This serves to draw attention to the project and encourage interested individuals to attend the presentation, and gives the members of the audience an opportunity to formulate questions beforehand. The researcher should aim to make the summary available a least 1 week prior to the scheduled presentation date.

Although the researching therapist may benefit in many ways from the process of presenting the proposal, the following points outline the main purposes of the presentation:

- To demonstrate to research colleagues that the therapist has gained an understanding of the background literature and relevant methodological issues which have resulted in the proposal of a project that will be worthy of the commitment of time and resources
- To give colleagues an opportunity to critically appraise the proposed methods and to make suggestions which can be incorporated into the project
- To give the therapist experience in verbal presentation of research material.

CONTENT

As proposal presentations are often only 10–15 minutes in duration only the most salient points from the written proposal should be given. The areas that should be included and guidelines for time allocation are given below. The exact content of each component and the order of their presentation will depend on the project. However, the presenter should aim to lead the audience in a logical fashion along a path which starts with the research question and finishes with a glimpse at the expected results and speculation on trends that may emerge. A brief summary may then be added to conclude the presentation and signal to the audience that they may begin the question period.

For a 10–5-minute presentation no more than 12–17 slides should be used (approximately one per minute, excluding the title and acknowledgement slides). The suggested areas to be covered are given in the following subsections. Examples of good slides and poor slides are provided in

Figures 6.1 to 6.5. Detailed information regarding slide or overhead transparency construction is provided in Chapter 19.

Title

The proposal presentation begins with a slide showing the title of the proposed study, the name of the investigator(s) and the name of the supervisor(s). This serves to focus the audience's attention on the topic and acknowledges the contribution of the supervisor or mentor in the development of the project.

Introduction or background

This should cover a brief review of the most relevant literature to give the audience some insight as to why the study is important and how it will contribute to knowledge in the area. This should lead to a statement of the problem and the main aim of the study.

Slides should consist of short phrases that summarize the main points. References which support these points may be included in parentheses, but as it is not the purpose of the presentation to dazzle the audience with the researcher's skills in searching the literature, only key references should be included. Approximately 20–30% of the presentation time should be allotted to this section.

Methods

This section forms the main focus of the presentation as it describes how the researcher proposes to answer the question. In light of this, approximately 30–40% of the time should be devoted to a description of the Methods.

In outlining the Methods the presenter should consider the background of the audience and give sufficient detail of the measurement procedures so that the majority can understand what is proposed. The following points should be included:

- Research design
- Research hypothesis(es), guiding questions

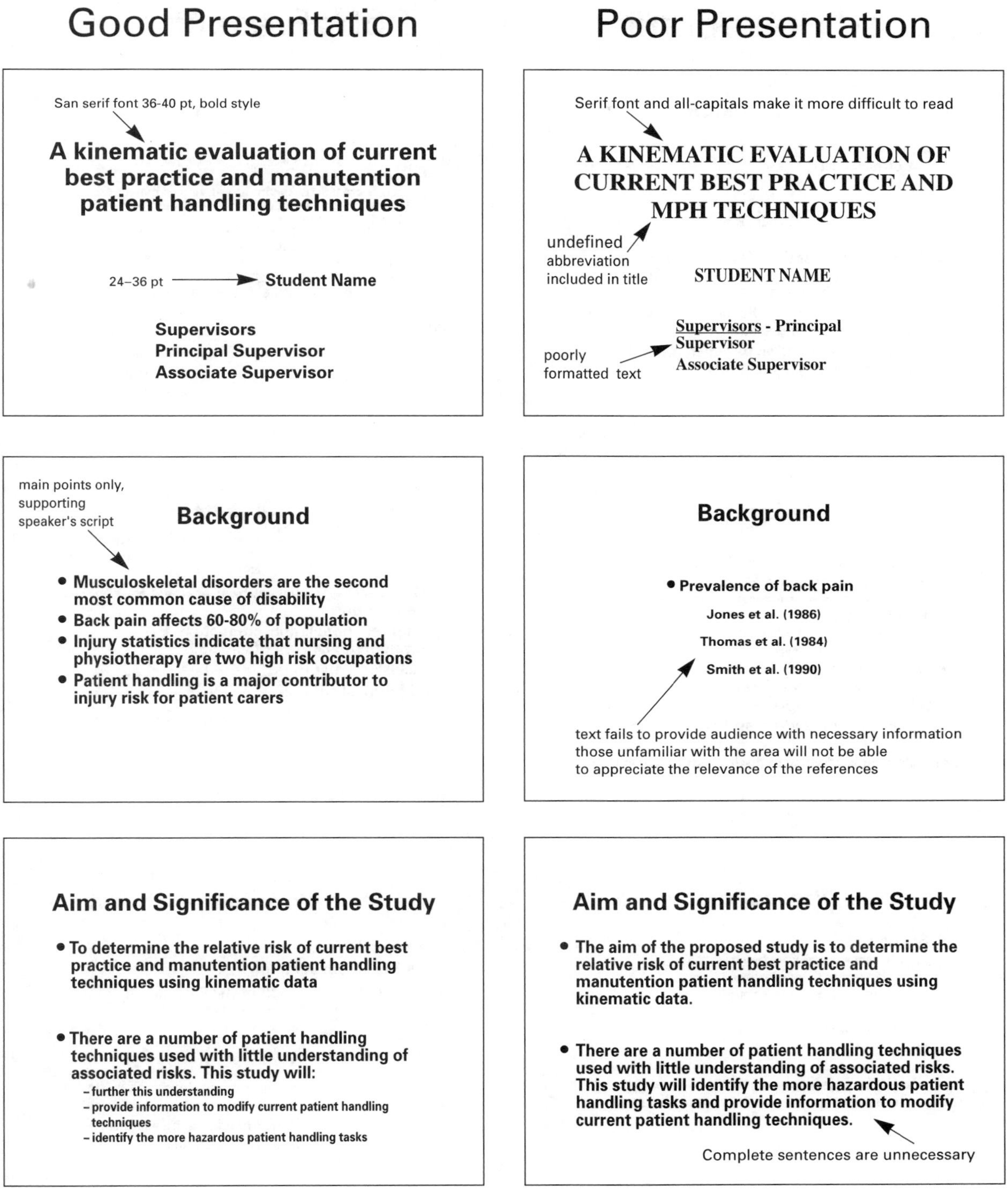

Good Presentation

Poor Presentation

San serif font 36-40 pt, bold style

A kinematic evaluation of current best practice and manutention patient handling techniques

24–36 pt ⟶ **Student Name**

Supervisors
Principal Supervisor
Associate Supervisor

Serif font and all-capitals make it more difficult to read

A KINEMATIC EVALUATION OF CURRENT BEST PRACTICE AND MPH TECHNIQUES

undefined abbreviation included in title

STUDENT NAME

poorly formatted text

Supervisors - Principal Supervisor
Associate Supervisor

main points only, supporting speaker's script

Background

- Musculoskeletal disorders are the second most common cause of disability
- Back pain affects 60-80% of population
- Injury statistics indicate that nursing and physiotherapy are two high risk occupations
- Patient handling is a major contributor to injury risk for patient carers

Background

- **Prevalence of back pain**

  Jones et al. (1986)

  Thomas et al. (1984)

  Smith et al. (1990)

text fails to provide audience with necessary information those unfamiliar with the area will not be able to appreciate the relevance of the references

Aim and Significance of the Study

- To determine the relative risk of current best practice and manutention patient handling techniques using kinematic data

- There are a number of patient handling techniques used with little understanding of associated risks. This study will:
  - further this understanding
  - provide information to modify current patient handling techniques
  - identify the more hazardous patient handling tasks

Aim and Significance of the Study

- The aim of the proposed study is to determine the relative risk of current best practice and manutention patient handling techniques using kinematic data.

- There are a number of patient handling techniques used with little understanding of associated risks. This study will identify the more hazardous patient handling tasks and provide information to modify current patient handling techniques.

Complete sentences are unnecessary

Figure 6.1 Example slides from a research proposal presentation illustrating a good presentation and a poor presentation Part 1

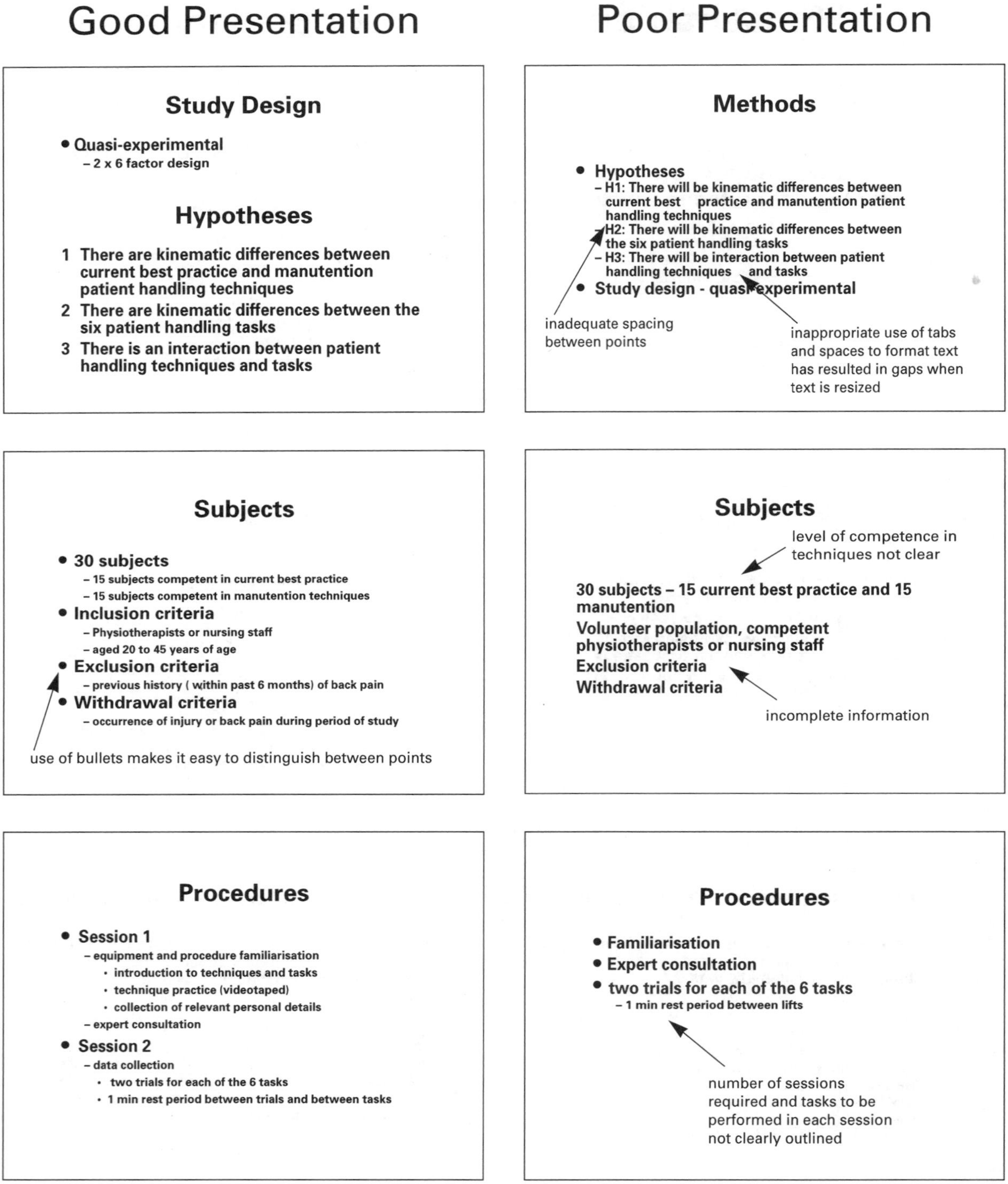

Figure 6.2 Example slides from a research proposal presentation illustrating a good presentation and a poor presentation Part 2

Good Presentation

Instrumentation

- Lumbar motion monitor

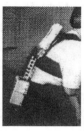

Variables

- Independent variables
  - patient handling technique
    - current best practice teachniques
    - manutention techniques
  - patient handling task
    - six common patient handling tasks
- Dependent variables
  - position of lumbar spine in three planes
  - angular velocity of lumbar spine in three planes
  - angular acceleration of lumbar spine in three planes

Controlled Variables

- standard patient weighing 55kg
- standard positioning of patient, subject and equipment
- consistency of patient handling technique

Poor Presentation

Instrumentation

- The lumbar motion monitor will be used to assess the position of each lumbar segment in space

although the description may be adequate a diagram provides the audience with a picture of the device and how it is applied to the subject

Variables

- patient handling technique - 2
- patient handling task - 6
- position, velocity, acceleration
  (of the lumbar spine in sagittal, coronal and transverse plane)

specification of number of levels is not clear

dependent and independent variables have not been not specified

Figure 6.3   Example slides from a research proposal presentation illustrating a good presentation and a poor presentation Part 3

Good Presentation

Poor Presentation

Special Ethical Issues

- Risk of injury will be reduced by ensuring:
  - adequate warmup
  - observation by a qualified therapist
  - maximum weight to be lifted of 55 kg
  - adequate rest between lifts

Ethics

- All subjects will sign an informed consent document
- Confidentiality will be preserved by
  - using subject ID number only
  - placing all data collection forms in a locked cupboard
  - restricting access to computer files
- Subjects are free to withdraw at any time without prejudice

This information can be considered as standard and does not need to be described to fellow researchers, inclusion takes valuable time from other areas of the proposal

Data Analysis

- Visual pattern analysis to assess data quality
- Data reduction to produce dependent variables
- Descriptive statistics
- Mixed model 2-way ANOVA
  - technique type = 2 levels
  - task type = 6 levels

Data Analysis

- data will be analysed using Excel and Statview 4.0
  - 2-way ANOVA

data quality testing and data reduction procedures have not been specified

Pilot Study

- Purpose
  - familiarise researcher with equipment
  - estimate time to complete testing sessions
  - identify unanticipated problems
- Method
  - 5 subjects
  - apply procedures for Session 1 and Session 2 on two separate days

Pilot Study

- 5 subjects will be tested

Figure 6.4 Example slides from a research proposal presentation illustrating a good presentation and a poor presentation Part 4

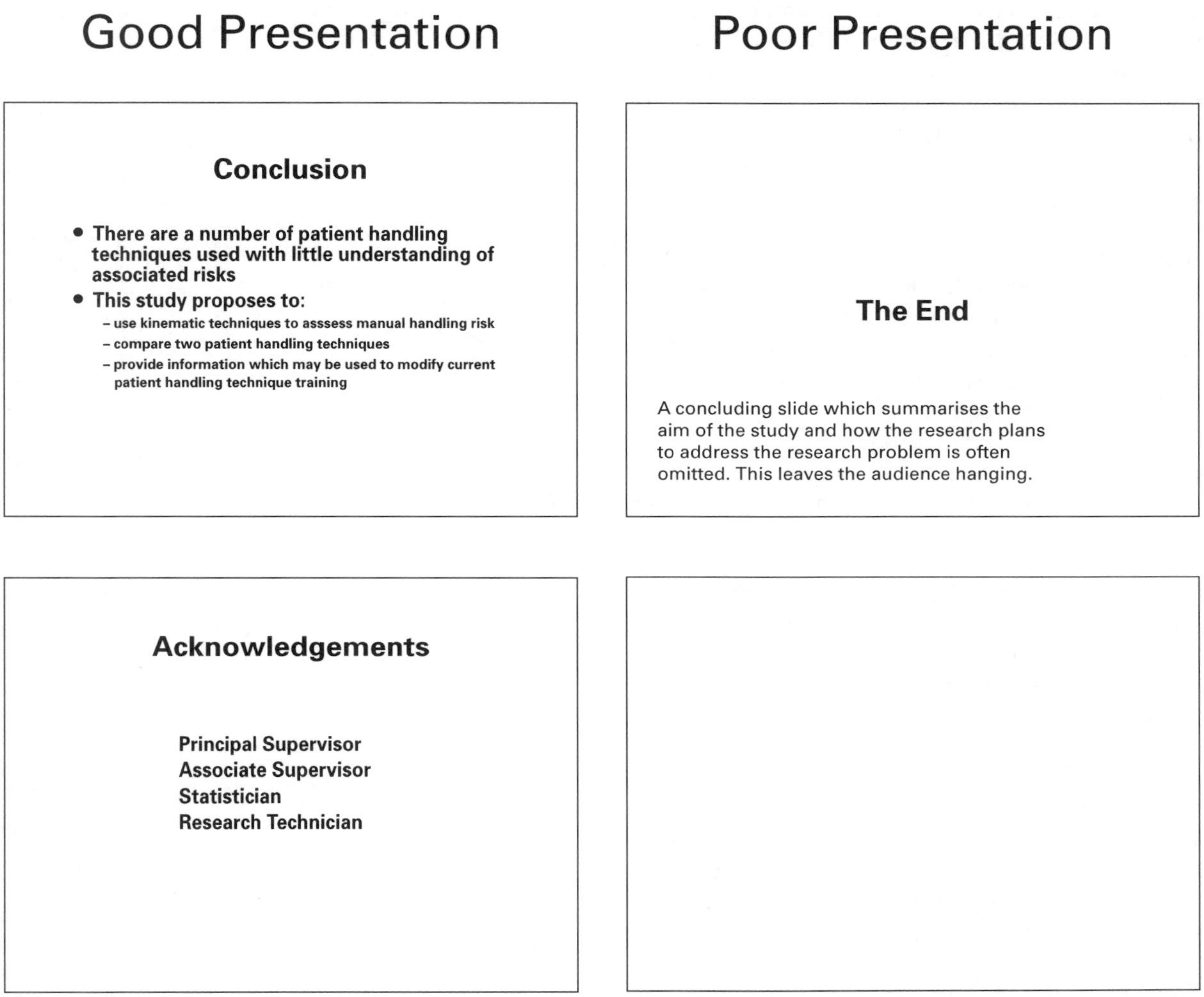

Good Presentation

Conclusion

- There are a number of patient handling techniques used with little understanding of associated risks
- This study proposes to:
  - use kinematic techniques to asssess manual handling risk
  - compare two patient handling techniques
  - provide information which may be used to modify current patient handling technique training

Acknowledgements

Principal Supervisor
Associate Supervisor
Statistician
Research Technician

Poor Presentation

The End

A concluding slide which summarises the aim of the study and how the research plans to address the research problem is often omitted. This leaves the audience hanging.

Figure 6.5 Example slides from a research proposal presentation illustrating a good presentation and a poor presentation Part 5

- Description of the subjects/participants, methods for recruiting, sample size, inclusion/exclusion/withdrawal criteria
- Variables: dependent, independent and extraneous (where appropriate)
- Procedures for testing or collecting data
- Any pilot studies which will be conducted; results of any preliminary testing already completed.

Owing to the time limitations it may not be possible to provide adequate details of some parts of the Methods; if the audience is attentive and interested this should spawn additional questions. These should be anticipated and the necessary resources prepared and organized to answer them effectively and efficiently.

Ethical considerations

This section need only include a brief statement indicating that the project will be scrutinized by the institution's ethics committee and that testing will not begin until approval has been obtained. Any special ethical problems may then be outlined in more detail, along with a description of how they will be managed.

Data analysis

If the study involves the collection of raw data requiring further reduction prior to analysis, the procedures which will be applied to the data should be outlined. The statistics that will be used to test the hypotheses or the procedures that will be used to answer the guiding questions should then be described.

Based on previous studies or pilot results, the therapist should give some indication of the expected results and may go on to speculate on trends that may emerge.

This portion of the presentation should be allotted 10–20% of the total time, depending on the complexity of the data reduction procedures that need to be outlined.

Conclusion

The presentation should be brought to a close with concluding remarks. These should restate the aim of the study, highlight how it proposes to meet this aim, and give implications for the potential findings.

Presenting the research proposal provides an important opportunity for the researching therapist to improve their communication skills and to receive feedback from research colleagues. With appropriate planning and rehearsal the experience should be rewarding.

7

Planning for ethical research

INTRODUCTION

Research projects should routinely acquire ethical clearance prior to the start of the study (Lo et al 1988). Most health and academic institutions have an established process for reviewing research projects. This generally involves an independent assessment of the study by an institutional ethics committee (IEC) to ensure that all ethical and legal obligations are met (Braddom 1990). Ethics committees operate under guidelines which have been developed since the Declaration of Helsinki in 1964, and refined through the Commissions for Human Rights and relevant national research funding agencies (e.g. the Australian National Health and Medical Research Council). From these sources guidelines for research using human subjects and for research using animals have been developed. This chapter will focus primarily on the ethical principles related to research involving human subjects.

Where research is undertaken outside an institution (or in an institution which does not have an IEC) the researching therapist should still seek to have the proposed project evaluated. In this situation the proposal may be evaluated by an existing IEC or by the therapist's professional association.

The purpose of this chapter is to describe the typical composition of an ethics committee, the basic principles for ethical research, guidelines for preparing ethics documentation and the nature of the review process in screening an application.

COMPOSITION OF ETHICS COMMITTEES

The purpose of the ethics committee is to evaluate the ethical, moral and legal implications of the study and to ensure that the interests of the community and of the institution are represented. In order to adequately represent the interests of the community most IECs seek to achieve a balance between the number of male and female members and to have individuals of different age groups if possible. Although the composition of an IEC may vary, the typical committee consists of the following: a laywoman, a layman, a medical graduate with research experience, a minister of religion or religious leader/elder and a lawyer (National Health and Medical Research Council 1982). At least one member of the committee must be someone who is not associated with the institution. The IEC is also able to co-opt members, who may provide specialist input when needed to resolve specific problems. The IEC will appoint a chairperson whose role is to conduct the meetings and oversee the activities of the committee, and additional support personnel are usually involved with managing correspondence and records.

ETHICAL PRINCIPLES RELATED TO RESEARCH INVOLVING HUMAN SUBJECTS

The basic tenet of ethical research is to preserve and protect the human dignity and rights of all subjects involved in a research project. The study must be recognized by peers and members of the community both to have value and benefit to the community at large, either in the present or in the future, and to have value beyond simply the 'need to know'.

During the review process the IEC evaluates the research proposal to determine whether sufficient consideration has been given to ethical issues in designing and presenting the project. In doing so several factors are considered. First, the description of the prospective subject population is evaluated to ensure that the sample will be appropriate with respect to the nature and goals of the project, and that subject selection will be conducted in a manner which ensures equity with regard to the potential risks and benefits. Characteristics of the population which may be considered include age range, gender, racial, ethnic or religious background, socioeconomic status, health or disability status, and position within an institution or culture. Special consideration is given to the involvement of individuals considered to be in a dependent or vulnerable position. These include children, residents of an institution (e.g. mentally or physically disabled individuals or elderly persons), wards of the state, prisoners, members of the armed services, those in teacher–student or doctor–patient relationships, pregnant women and fetuses. The size of the sample is also evaluated to ensure that a sufficient but not excessive number of subjects will be included to meet the aims of the study.

Secondly, the potential risks and benefits are identified and a risk–benefit analysis is performed. A risk is defined as any potential harm, including discomfort, burden, inconvenience or injury, that may occur as a result of participation in the study (Prentice & Purtilo 1993), and may be categorized as physical, psychological, social or economic. Both immediate and latent or delayed risks should be identified, as should any factors that might increase the potential risk for certain subjects (e.g. pregnant women). Once identified, each risk is then evaluated to determine whether it can be considered to be minimal (i.e. the consequences of participation are not greater in and of themselves than that which might be encountered in daily life or during a routine procedure) or more than minimal. In research, the ethical principle of maleficence (do no harm) guides the consideration of risk.

In health research, procedures are specifically evaluated to determine whether they are considered to be 'invasive' and thus carry a specific risk. This notion applies as much to physically invasive procedures (e.g. taking a blood sample) as to procedures or questions which may be psychologically, socially or emotionally invasive.

The evaluation of the potential benefits involves the assessment of perceived benefits, both to the subject directly and to the community at large. In research the ethical principle of beneficence (the act of promoting good for others) guides the consideration of benefits.

Once the potential risks and benefits have been identified and classified, a risk–benefit analysis will be performed. During the review process the researcher must be able to represent to the satisfaction of the IEC that the merit (benefits) of the investigation outweigh the risks of participation. Where there are stated risks or costs, it must be shown that these can be anticipated adequately and their probability or consequence reduced as much as is reasonably possible. For example, the probability of pain and injury from maximal exercise testing could be reduced by excluding vulnerable subjects, and the consequences of the risk of cardiac arrest during maximal exercise testing could be reduced by having a medical attendant and resuscitation equipment on standby. Similarly, there may be an important benefit to other groups in society arising from the participation of the volunteers in the proposed investigation, even where the subjects may not experience this benefit directly. The aspect of risk versus benefit is one of the most important 'watchdog' roles of the IEC and must be anticipated by the researcher when preparing the research proposal.

Thirdly, the process of obtaining informed consent is evaluated. For consent to be legally and ethically valid it must meet certain requirements:

- It must be voluntary, obtained without deceit, coercion, fraud or the intervention of any element of force or constraint
- The person involved must have the legal capacity to give consent
- The person involved must have sufficient knowledge of the procedures or activities involved, and understand the implications of giving consent.

Finally, the investigators' qualifications may be reviewed to ensure that they have the appropriate qualifications/licensure to carry out the specified procedures, and that adequate facilities and equipment will be available to conduct the research.

To assist the members of the IEC in their evalu-ation the following sections of the research proposal should be clearly identifiable and contain adequate information as described.

THE INFORMED CONSENT DOCUMENT

As research involving humans is often an imposed activity, however benign, there is an obligation on the investigator to obtain informed consent from each subject prior to undertaking the study. Each subject must be able to make an informed judgement about their participation which is based on written documentation provided by the researcher. This must provide a clear statement of the purpose of the investigation and what is required of the subjects in terms of their time, activity, travel, special tests, etc. There must be a full disclosure of what personal information will be sought, and the nature and form of this information and the proposed use of the collected data must be stated.

At the time of granting consent, the subject must acknowledge the significance of the information presented to them, and must be provided with a signed copy of the consent document(s). The legal implications of this must be noted, as any future action could test the adequacy of such information. To protect both the subject and the researcher, written consent should be obtained from all subjects and filed appropriately. In the case of questionnaires, completion and return of the document is considered to indicate consent (NB: a statement to this effect should be placed on the front of the questionnaire).

Subjects must give written, informed consent before participating in a study. The consent form must be dated and include the signatures and full names of the subject, the researcher(s) and, where possible, a witness. In the case of a child, the full information should be given to the parent(s) or guardian and as much information as is reasonable provided for the child. Children should be given the chance to sign the form as well as their parent(s) or legal advocate; the latter must sign the form if the child is below the legal age as deemed appropriate by the state. There may be occasions when a subject is unable to read the consent form: every attempt should be made to overcome this (e.g. enlarging text, translating into another language). If the subject is still unable to read the form then the form must be read to them. Where the subject is physically unable to sign, other methods of consent (verbal or non-verbal assent) may be considered valid if witnessed by a legal advocate (carer/relative) for the subject.

Generally the informed consent document consists of two components: the participant information sheet and the consent form. Although the elements that make up the informed consent document are reasonably consistent, some variation may be found between different institutions regarding the organization of its contents.

As the purpose of the consent document is to inform and guide the negotiations with the prospective participant, the language and style should reflect this intent. By writing the consent document in the second person (using the pronoun 'you'), the researcher conveys the sentiment that the participant is being dealt with on an individual basis and that they are being given the opportunity to make a choice. The language used should be simple enough to be understood by the least educated or worldly of the prospective subjects, for this reason technical terms and professional jargon must be avoided; if such a term must be included it should be defined.

The following sections provide a guide to the elements that should be included in the informed consent document. It is recommended that subheadings are used to distinguish the various elements, as this increases the readability of the document for both the subject and the members of the IEC. A sample of an informed consent document is provided in Appendix A.

Title

The title on the consent document may need to be different from the title given on the research proposal, so that it may be understood by the prospective participants and by the lay reviewers on the IEC. The format of the title is similar to that described for the research proposal, where only the initial word is capitalized. Abbreviations should not be included in the title. For example, a

research proposal entitled *Kinetic and kinematic investigation of the translatory and rotatory movement patterns used by individuals with spinal cord injury during transferring* may be rewritten as *Transferring and reaching in individuals with spinal cord injury.*

Purpose of the project

A brief explanation of the purpose of the study should be included in order to help the prospective participant to assess the importance of the study in relation to their own values. This explanation should give a clear rationale for undertaking the study, why it is important and the reason(s) for selecting the particular subject. This section may be introduced with an invitation to the subject, for example: *You are asked to participate in a study designed to determine which of two treatments is best for the treatment of tennis elbow, a condition from which you suffer.*

Procedures

The procedures section should include a description of the study design (including the method of assignment to groups where appropriate); a description of each procedure that is to be applied to, or activity to be performed by, the subject and how often it will be performed; identification of the individual(s) who will perform the procedures or interact with the subject; where and when the research will be conducted; and an estimate of the time commitment required of the subject. Where necessary, a statement should be included concerning any medications or other substances, foods, therapeutic regimens or other activities that are contraindicated, disallowed, or which require modification.

For the description of the procedures, full details must be given in terms that can be easily understood. For example, if oxygen saturation is to be measured using a pulse oximeter and finger sensor, in lay terms this could be written as follows: *The amount of oxygen in your blood will be measured by placing a small sensor on your index finger. The sensor shines a light through your finger and the amount of light which passes through depends on the level of oxygen in your blood.*

If the subject is a patient, it must be clearly stated which procedures are part of normal care and which are for the purposes of the study only.

Risks, discomforts and benefits

This section should outline both the immediate and long-term risks and benefits of the procedures applied during the course of the study. The disclosure of risks should be evaluated based on what a reasonably prudent subject might wish to know, and the risks should neither be understated nor overstated. If the procedures carry any risk of discomfort an estimate of the probability, severity, average duration and reversibility of such discomfort should be given.

Alternatives to participation

If the efficacy of a treatment intervention is being studied, all reasonable alternatives to this treatment must be outlined. This section may be omitted if it does not apply.

Financial obligations or compensation

All financial obligations related to participation in the study (e.g. transportation costs) or any costs for services provided (e.g. medications, laboratory tests, physician or therapist fees) should be outlined. Any economic incentives or rewards for participation should also be clearly stated, including any conditions that apply to the receipt of remuneration.

Confidentiality

This section should include details of how the information or samples obtained from the subject will be handled, stored and disposed of, and how the subject's confidentiality will be maintained (see discussion on p. 49–50).

Request for more information

This section consists of a written offer to provide the subject with more information at any time regarding the study or their rights as a participant. To facilitate this, contact details for the researcher and a representative of the institution in which the research is performed should be included in the consent document.

Refusal or withdrawal

The consent document should include a disclaimer which states that the subject may refuse to participate in the study and that they may withdraw their consent to participate at any time (including after all data have been collected), without prejudice to themselves (or others) and without penalty or fear of implications for their future care or management. (NB: If a subject withdraws their consent after the data have been collected their data and all related material must be destroyed.)

Consent statement

As the consent document is a contract between the researcher and the subject it must include a statement indicating that the signatures on the document certify the subject's voluntary and informed consent to participate in the study.

Signatures

Dated signatures of the participant (or their parent, guardian or legal advocate if they are a minor or unable to give consent) and the researcher are the concluding elements of the consent document. Where possible, the signature of a witness (who is not the researcher) is also recommended.

SPECIFIC CONFIDENTIALITY ISSUES

In most research situations the researcher cannot guarantee anonymity (anonymous questionnaires being the exception), but should take the necessary steps to preserve participant confidentiality. This is accomplished by ensuring that:

- Any information recorded from subjects is

kept in a secure location with restricted access, usually reserved for the investigators
- Any information, photographs or recordings obtained in connection with the study that could identify the subject will be disclosed only with the subject's permission
- At the completion of the project all data are archived in a secure location and destroyed at the end of the specified retention period.

To preserve confidentiality each subject should be assigned a unique identifying code on entry to the study, and this should be used to mark subsequent data collection forms and computer files.

If a subject is to be recorded audiovisually, this must be disclosed in the consent form. If tapes, videos or photographs are taken, the subject should know who will keep them, who will have access and how they will be used (e.g. for presentations or publications relating to the research).

In some studies one-way mirrors may be used to enable discreet observation. If so, subjects must be informed of this and told who the observers will be.

Photographs of a subject should only be used in publications or presentations if they have given written, informed consent prior to the taking of the photograph (see Appendix B for an example consent form). To preserve anonymity (in publications and presentations), some journal editors require that facial and other identifying features be covered or obliterated in the reproduction.

THE REVIEW PROCESS

The procedures for obtaining ethical clearance are usually clearly documented for each institution. The researcher should obtain the necessary guidelines and forms from each institution involved in the project. Specific details regarding the structure and length of the proposal should be observed, and the procedures and likely time involved in the review process should be noted. Commonly, the guidelines will require that the researcher submit multiple copies of the research proposal to the IEC. These may then be distrib-

Hazard 7.1

For some institutions the ethics review process may take several weeks or months owing to the timing and frequency of IEC meetings. This can result in significant delays as subject recruitment and data collection cannot be commenced until approval is received

uted to the various members of the IEC for review before the next meeting. The schedule of such meetings should be obtained so that the submission can be prepared accordingly. If the IEC is satisfied that all of the necessary criteria have been met, a document signifying approval will be issued and the study may begin. If this is not the case, the submission may be returned to the researcher accompanied by a request for certain issues to be addressed. The proposal may then need to be resubmitted to the committee. Occasionally the chairperson may approve the revised proposal on behalf of the committee.

If the proposal is being submitted for external funding, and formal approval cannot be obtained prior to the submission, provisional clearance may be given by the chairperson of the IEC. Funding agencies may then require that the formal approval be forwarded before the funds are released.

Ethics approval is generally granted for a specified period only, and may need to be renewed during the course of the study. The IEC may also require regular reporting (usually annually) and notification of any significant changes to the study that may have ethical implications. A final report on the research may also be requested by the IEC. This usually documents the progress to completion of the study, and describes the number of subjects recruited, reasons for any withdrawals, any adverse reactions (physical or emotional) to the intervention or testing, and steps taken in response to these problems. If publications have been submitted or published from the study, they should be appended to this report.

When planning any research project, regardless of whether IEC approval is required, the researcher should follow the ethical principles and processes outlined in this chapter. By so doing the ethical, moral and legal implications of the study can be considered and appropriate actions can be taken before it begins. The researcher should also be mindful of the ethical principles throughout the study and when reporting the findings.

Acknowledgements
The authors are grateful to Associate Professor Rosemary Coates for assistance with material for this chapter.

REFERENCES

Braddom C L 1990 The ethics of research. American Journal of Physical Medicine and Rehabilitation 69: 170–171

Lo B, Feigal D, Cummins S, Hulley S B 1988 Addressing ethical issues. In: Hulley S B, Cummings S R (eds) Designing clinical research. Williams & Wilkins, Baltimore

National Health and Medical Research Council 1982 Ethics in medical research: report of the NH & MRC working party on ethics in medical research. Australian Government Publishing Service, Canberra

National Health and Medical Research Council 1987 Statement on human experimentation. Australian Government Publishing Service, Canberra

Prentice E D, Purtilo R B 1993 The use and protection of human and animal subjects. In: Bork C (ed) Research in Physical Therapy. J B Lippincott Company, Philadelphia, 37–56

Applying for research funding

The aim of applying for funding is to obtain the resources required to perform the desired research. Applying for research funding usually requires a considerable expenditure of time and energy, so if the resources can be acquired without formal application to funding organizations the researcher may choose to invest their time in other aspects of the research process. However, many research projects benefit from, or require, funding. To enhance the researcher's chances of success when applying for funding, this chapter describes the funding process and a typical grant application.

THE RESEARCH FUNDING PROCESS

The research funding process is like a futures market. The researching therapist is a seller: the research proposal is really a promise to deliver specified knowledge (the product) at a stated time in the future. The funding organization is the buyer and is interested in buying knowledge. This process is illustrated in Figure 8.1.

To be successful in acquiring funding the researcher must understand the market, provide a quality product at a reasonable price and find an interested buyer with the capital to buy.

The buyers

The funding sources which are the potential buyers of the therapist's research include professional societies and associations, government departments or institutes, charities and commer-

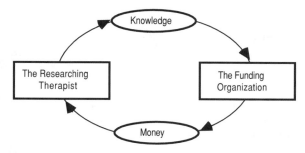

Figure 8.1 The research funding market

cial organizations. Each type of organization will require a different type of grant application, targeted to their interests and requirements.

Potential funding sources can be identified by noting advertisements in mass media and professional and institutional newsletters, noting acknowledgements in articles and presentations, asking colleagues and contacting university research offices.

The therapist needs to be able to answer two pertinent questions about any funding organization:

- Is it interested in the knowledge the research project will provide?
- Does it provide funds of sufficient magnitude?

To answer these and later more detailed questions, documentation supplied by each organization specifically on grants and annual reports, should be carefully reviewed. The organization's grants officer is usually able to provide considerable insight into what is important to the organization and how competitive the process is. This information will be useful in enabling the researcher to eliminate unlikely prospects.

Funding organizations differ in the degree of rigour they expect and in the amount of competition for their funds. Often, prestigious government-funded organizations have very high standards and are extremely competitive. For example, an organization applied to by one of the authors has a 10% funding rate after substandard applications are removed. This means that only one out of every 10 good applications will be funded. Professional associations, charitable trusts and commercial organizations tend to

place less weight on scientific rigour and more emphasis on the relevance of the topic to their aims. In both cases, the difference between a good application and a successful one may be how well the goals of the institution have been addressed.

The money

Research grants are typically in cash, but can also be in kind, such as the use of equipment or time release. Cash grants can either be for an individual or for a project.

Scholarships (usually for research towards a graduate degree) and fellowships (usually for post-degree research) are available for individuals to perform research. These may provide enough resources to give a therapist time to plan, perform and communicate a research project by providing an income. Scholarships are usually around half a clinical salary, whereas fellowships are closer to a typical clinical or academic salary. Both usually have small allowances for thesis preparation and some provide assistance for travel to conferences. Competition for government-funded scholarships and fellowships is usually quite fierce, with the therapies being potentially at a disadvantage by not having the high undergraduate marks of pure sciences nor the name of medicine. There are some scholarships and fellowships specifically for therapies or particular study areas, and these may be more fruitful for the researching therapist to explore.

Project grants range from small 'seeding' grants to large grants for collaborative international projects. Project grants do not provide funds for an individual, but rather for a specified project. For the new researcher the likelihood of success will probably be greatest with seeding grants, as there will not be the expectation of a substantial research track record. Similarly, professional associations, charitable trusts and commercial organizations are more likely to fund a new researcher than are the government research organizations. For large grants with budgets covering a number of staff over a number of years, a significant track record of grants and publications will usually be required.

The focus for this chapter is on project grant

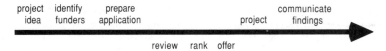

Figure 8.2 The research funding process

applications, although most principles will also apply to applications for scholarships and fellowships.

The product

The 'product' that funding organizations buy is knowledge. Thus the grant application needs to clearly state the outcomes so that the funder can see what they are buying. The document conveying this information, the grant application, must be of high presentation quality. Similarly, the price of the project must be within the organization's capabilities and suited to the significance of the information to be delivered.

The sellers

Although sometimes difficult, it is useful to glean information about other 'sellers' and their 'products'. Many funding organizations prepare annual reports with details of which projects have been funded, the amount granted, what the projects were about and who performed them. This information can be used to see what types of projects and research teams have been successful in the past.

The process

Assuming a project idea has already been developed, the process of applying for funding begins by identifying and becoming familiar with potential funding organizations. Using the information from and about each funding organization, a grant application is prepared and submitted according to the organization's requirements. The researcher then waits while the application is reviewed and – hopefully – shortlisted. They may then be called to an interview as part of the review process.

Following review, suitable applications are usually ranked, with the most highly ranked projects being funded, working down the ranking until all the funds are committed. The lucky researcher is then offered a certain amount of funding and usually signs a contract to perform the research in return for that specified amount. They then perform the research and provide progress and final reports as required. Finally, the researcher usually communicates the findings to the broader community. Figure 8.2 illustrates this process, with activities by the researcher above the arrow and those of the funding agency below.

As with the preparation of a research proposal (see Chapter 5), the process of applying for research funds is facilitated by assistance from experts. The researching therapist can improve their chances of success by using experienced colleagues to help with the development of the research idea, the preparation of the grant application, the preparation for any interview and in re-evaluation of the application following the outcome of the review process.

Developing a research idea into a well conceptualized proposal is explained in previous chapters, and page 55 provides details on the preparation and content of a grant application.

Not all funding organizations use an interview as part of the application review process, but for those who do this is an excellent opportunity for the researcher to sell their project. In preparation for the interview the researching therapist should first refamiliarize themselves with the application, as several months may have elapsed since preparing it, and secondly, prepare a brief summary of the research (what will be done, why it is important and what the outcomes will be). It is useful to ask experienced colleagues who are unfamiliar with the project to review the application and run a mock interview, as it is much better to identify inadequacies before the interview with the funding organization.

Review interview panels typically have a number of members from different backgrounds. The researcher should therefore prepare to answer specific questions in detail (e.g. on sample size selection) but be able to talk in plain language during most of the interview, so that each panel member can understand the need for the research and the quality of the proposed study. It is often useful to have a few photographs, diagrams or graphs to illustrate key points. Time is limited in interviews, so it is important to focus on the main points and not waste time on trivia. Chapter 19, although not directed at the interview situation, has suggestions which will improve the delivery of information in the interview and the impression created by the researching therapist.

Whether or not the application is successful, the researcher should endeavour to learn from the experience by acquiring feedback from the funding organization on the strengths and weaknesses of the application and interview.

The final phase of the research process is the communication of the findings. This is an integral part of the process and is seen as an ethical responsibility of the researching therapist. Successful publication of the findings of funded research (with acknowledgement of the funding agency) will also enhance the therapist's chances of further funding.

Key Points 8.1

Begin with a well developed idea

Carefully evaluate the goals of the likely funding organizations

Be pedantic in following funding organization's application requirements

Prepare for interview by rehearsal with experienced colleagues

Obtain feedback on application regardless of outcome

If successful, ensure quality publications are produced

THE GRANT APPLICATION

The grant application is the main selling tool available to the researching therapist. It is critical that this is prepared with flawless professionalism and with the utmost attention to detail, in the style of the funding organization. One useful tip is to try to use the terminology of the organization as much as possible, as this will enable the organization's reviewers to easily see how the project fits with its aims.

Research grant applications typically require information on the project's title, the research team, the project, the background, the research aim, research plan, expected outcomes and their implications, ethics approval, details of other support and details of the requested budget. An explanation of each of these items and suggestions for their content are given in the following paragraphs.

The project title

The title of the project is very important and should be written so that it is clearly of direct interest to the funding organization. It should also be written in the language style expected by the organization. For example, the grant application for a project which will evaluate the validity of a simulated driving assessment for predicting the return to driving of clients with head injuries could be titled *Returning safely to driving* for an application to a charitable society, or *The predictive validity of a virtual driving simulator for patients with parietal lobe head injuries following motor vehicle accidents* for an application to a national medical research council.

The research team

Project grant applications typically come from research teams. Aspects of the team which are likely to impress the funding organization include evidence of their ability to do research (a track record of grants and related publications), appropriate discipline qualifications, appropriate mix of qualifications and employment with respected research organizations.

Multidisciplinary teams are often seen as desirable as they provide the range of skills necessary for many research projects.

Care should also be taken that the team meets the requirements of the funding organization. For example, some organizations require the chief investigator to be from a particular discipline and to *not* be a tertiary student.

Most funding organizations require team members to sign confirming their commitment to the project. In addition, a research officer in the institution which will manage the grant usually reviews and signs the application prior to its being sent to the funding organization. (Time should be allocated for the institutional review so that the application still meets the funding organization's deadlines.)

Background to the project

Space is usually tightly controlled and limited in research grant applications. Thus the background to the project, despite starting from a broad base, must quickly narrow in focus. This section has similar requirements to the Introduction in a research proposal (see Chapter 5, p. 28). The research problem needs to be briefly reviewed and its significance clearly portrayed. This section should convince the funding organization that something desperately needs to be done about this important problem. The research plan and expected outcomes sections should convince the organization that this particular project is the best way to address the problem. The language style needs to be targeted to the expectations of the organization. A non-personal, technical style with frequent reference to publications in esteemed journals may be appropriate for some organizations, whereas a more personal or authoritative style may be suitable for others.

The research aim

The research aim should be clear, flow logically from the background to the project and meet a need of the funding organization. This section is sometimes called research objectives or hypotheses. Organizations that request the latter heading usually have a preference for highly controlled quantitative designs, and consequently it may be difficult for projects which do not have a hypothesis to obtain funding.

The research plan

Most grant application forms do not provide sufficient space to give all the details of the methods provided in a comprehensive research proposal. However, sufficient detail must be provided to convince the reviewer that the researcher plans to use an appropriate design and understands the methods sufficiently to explain them well. Concise descriptions of the design, participants, data to be collected, procedures and analysis should be given. Many organizations also require a project time plan, with key milestones noted. Even if this is not required, a clear task by time graph (see Chapter 11, p. 78) suggests competent project management skills.

Expected outcomes

The expected outcomes is a critical section of the application. It explains what knowledge the funding organization is buying and what are the implications of that knowledge. New researchers should not be tempted to claim too much, as the experienced reviewers will recognize that more is being claimed than can be delivered and probably recommend that the project not be funded owing to researcher inexperience or unrealistic expectations.

When writing the expected outcomes and their implications the researcher should try to target the goals of the organization. This can be made very explicit by using the relevant terminology.

Ethics

For research involving humans or animals, funding organizations will usually require confirmation from a recognized ethics committee that the project meets ethical requirements (see Chapter 7). Sometimes organizations will review applications pending final ethical approval.

Other support

Most grant application forms ask what other assistance is either already available or has been requested, including applications for similar support from other funding organizations. It may also include offers of support already negotiated, for example time release for the therapist. Showing that some support has already been provided demonstrates that others are convinced of the project's merit.

Budget

Preparation of the budget should be relatively easy when a good project proposal has already been prepared (see Chapter 5). Two components are usually required: a detailed breakdown on expected expenditure and a justification for each expenditure item.

The breakdown of expenditure is typically into categories, such as personnel, equipment, travel, consumables and other.

To calculate personnel costs, the time required of staff and the level of competence needed must be estimated. To assist with the estimation of time required, the description of research tasks developed for the proposal can be used. Thus subject recruitment could be estimated to take 5 days, equipment piloting a further 5 days, and so on. These can then be summed to give the overall project requirements, allowing for some additional organization time. The level of staff competence may be that of an undergraduate student or a qualified and experienced clinician, and will need to be justified in terms of the tasks to be performed. The level of competence will determine the level of pay. Some organizations require staff costs to include overheads, such as workers' compensation, superannuation and leave entitlements. (Exact salary and overhead cost rates can be acquired from human resources departments.) Some funding organizations will not provide funds for the chief investigator, only for research assistants. Further, many applications require estimates of how much time each member of the research team will spend on the project. In both situations it should be made very clear what the funding applied for covers, and what staff time is already being provided.

Equipment requests in budgets must be seen to be essential to the project and include only equipment which is not normally available to the therapist. Thus a study measuring trunk movement could easily justify an electrogoniometer, but justification for a desktop computer would be more difficult.

Some funding organizations will pay for researcher and participant travel associated with the project, and some will even pay for the researcher to attend a conference to present the findings.

Consumables include paper, printing, postage, digital storage media, electrodes, disposable mouthpieces and telecommunication costs. Projects requiring the distribution of multipaged questionnaires to many subjects may have a large consumable cost, whereas other projects may have very small expected costs. The opportunity to claim for other miscellaneous requirements is usually provided. This could include paying for diagnostic tests, legal advice or archiving of data. Table 8.1 illustrates a budget for a biomechanical study of risk in lifting tasks.

Often a high level of infrastructure support is expected from the researcher, such that computing, local travel and consumables will not be funded. Also, institutions where the researching therapist is employed or enrolled may take a cut of the grant.

Researchers should provide realistic budgets, remembering that peers with research budget experience will probably be assessing the costs. There is a disturbing trend for capital-restricted funding organizations to try to offer more grants by cutting, say, 20% off all budgets. In an ideal world researchers would return such an offer saying that the research is not possible with anything but the full budget. However, a more likely (but still principled) response is to accept the funding and state what reductions will be made to the project to keep it within the reduced budget.

Each item detailed in the budget should be justified with clear and convincing reasons why it is necessary for the project to succeed, as shown in the following example:

Table 8.1 Example of grant application budget for a biomechanical study on lifting

Budget	Total ($)
Personnel	
0.5 Research assistant level 2.1 salary for 12 months	12,943
Overhead costs at 11% (superannuation, workers comp.)	1,424
Subtotal	14,367
Equipment	
WATBAK biomechanical analysis software	1,200
Scaffolding and hardboard	450
Subtotal	1,650
Travel	
Return airfare to national research conference	738
2 nights' accommodation @ $114	228
Subtotal	966
Consumables	
2 x 600k optical digital storage disks	600
Photocopying, printing and paper	100
Subtotal	700
Other	
Remuneration for subjects	2,460
Subtotal	2,460
Total	**20,143**

To evaluate the hypothesis, estimates of lumbar compression forces are required. The WATBAK biomechanical software analysis program is the only commercially available program for the analysis of static loads on the lumbar spine which does not assume an extensor capability for intra-abdominal pressure (the latter being widely reported as invalid in recent years).

Hazard 8.1

Asking for too little

Promising too much

Applying to organization not interested in topic or philosophically opposed to approach taken

Wrong time and place

This chapter has provided an overview of the typical process of applying for research project funding and provided suggestions for the preparation and content of a grant application.

Further Reading

Dreher M 1994 Qualitative research methods from a reviewer's perspective. In: Morse J (ed) Critical issues in qualitative research methods. Sage Publications, Thousand Oaks, USA, pp. 281–297

Richards L 1993 Writing a qualitative thesis or grant application. In: Beattie K (ed) Where's your research profile? A resource book for academics. Union of Australian College of Academics, Melbourne, pp. 30–44

3

Performing research

SECTION CONTENTS

Working as part of a team

Research is seldom undertaken by an individual working in isolation. More commonly, a number of individuals, sometimes from different disciplines, work together on a research project. The extent of involvement of each team member may vary, and this will have a bearing on the ranking of the authors when the research findings are communicated (see Chapter 16, p. 128). In some instances research is performed by a group of undergraduate or postgraduate students under the supervision of a member of academic staff. Such research generally forms the assessed component of a unit or course of study, and all students receive the same mark for the work. In this case it is especially important that the workload is shared equally.

There are many benefits of working as a team. These include dividing the workload, sharing the highs and lows of the experience, being able to have informed discussions about the research and having help to resolve problems (e.g. technical difficulties with instrumentation). However, working with others may at times be frustrating. Sometimes this is due to the different work practices of the individuals. The following suggestions and guidelines are intended to assist with the team research process. Not all will be applicable in every situation: some will only apply to students working together on a project.

THE FIRST MEETING

The following paragraphs outline the importance of the first meeting and cover the allocation of roles to individual team members, work habits, team rules and meeting schedules and record keeping.

At the first meeting it may be helpful to identify individuals with expertise in a particular area. For example, one person may have a strong background in statistical methods, and another may be very familiar with some of the instrumentation to be used. It may be appropriate to assign particular tasks to individuals based on their skills. When the team consists of members from different disciplines, the areas of expertise and the appropriate roles may be immediately evident. Sometimes an individual's strengths or weaknesses do not become apparent until the research is under way and therefore it may be necessary to renegotiate roles at regular intervals.

Each individual should discuss their approach to work, in particular to meeting deadlines. Some individuals work better under stress and leave tasks until very close to the deadline. Others always complete tasks well ahead of time. It is helpful if team members declare their approach to deadlines at the first meeting, as this enables differences to be incorporated into the teamwork process and may be used to obtain agreement on how achieving deadlines will be managed.

It is extremely useful for the team to discuss what is likely to make the team work well together and what is likely to be unproductive. From this discussion it may be appropriate to establish some rules of conduct for the team, which all members agree to abide by until the team decides otherwise. Any such rules must be documented and used for future reference when necessary. One suggestion is that all information relating to the project (e.g. rules of conduct and minutes of meetings) is recorded in the project file, which is kept by one team member, and that this is referred to during discussions (see Chapter 11, p. 74–75, and Chapter 12, p. 80–84).

There should be a general plan for the frequency of meetings. This may vary at different stages in the research, but it is generally unproductive if long periods elapse between meetings. The team should decide who will take responsibility for organizing a venue, gathering items for the agenda, chairing the meeting and taking minutes. Ideally these tasks should be shared and the roles may be alternated between team members.

Minutes of all meetings should be recorded in the project file. The record should include the names of those present and any apologies, a list of the issues discussed, the actions arising, the person(s) responsible for executing the actions and timelines. Each member should receive a copy of the minutes and these should be referred to at subsequent meetings, so that the team can keep a record of the actions implemented.

MUTUAL RESPECT

Problems will arise if team members do not respect each other's time and (where applicable) that of the project supervisor. Showing mutual respect means attending all meetings, arriving on time and staying for the duration unless prior commitments are declared in advance. It also means allowing each person in the team to have an input to the meetings and not allowing one person to dominate.

For successful teamwork each member must make every possible effort to complete assigned tasks by agreed deadlines. Where this appears unlikely, the individual should notify other team members early to enlist assistance.

WORKLOAD SHARING

The equal sharing of the workload is a very important issue in the context of research performed by students. (It should of course be noted that written output is not the only measure of work.) To keep a check on the amount of work undertaken by each individual, it may be appropriate for all team members (in confidence) to rate their own contribution and that of every other team member. An example of a workload evaluation form is given in Figure 9.1.

Written comments should be made to justify these evaluations. If such a method is adopted then it is recommended that an assessment of workload is carried out at appropriate intervals throughout the research process, for example after the research proposal has been submitted

	Major contribution	Some contribution	Little contribution
Leadership and direction	☐	☐	☐
Ideas, suggestions, contributions to group discussions	☐	☐	☐
Information gathering and interpreting	☐	☐	☐
Data collection	☐	☐	☐
Data analysis	☐	☐	☐
Report writing	☐	☐	☐

Figure 9.1   Criteria for workload evaluation for contribution to a research project (adapted from Gibbs et al 1986)

and upon completion of the project. Inequalities in workload may be dealt with by open discussion with all team members or in consultation with the project supervisor. Workload assessments should be used when deciding the ranking of authors on communications (see Chapter 16, p. 128).

CONFLICT RESOLUTION

Disagreements and conflicts are inevitable and team members will react to these in different ways. The ability to negotiate is a fundamental and necessary skill for conflict resolution. This skill can be acquired (Maddux 1988). Learning to manage conflict is not only necessary for effective teamwork in research, but also in many aspects of professional life. As with most 'disorders', early intervention is the most effective treatment: problems should be addressed as soon as they appear. Honest and open discussion is necessary and, where possible, a compromise should be agreed upon. When the team is unable to resolve conflicts the assistance of an appropriate person should be sought. This may be the academic supervisor of the project, the project supervisor, an academic staff member, a manager (e.g. head of department) or a counsellor.

REFERENCE

Maddux R B 1988 Successful negotiation: effective "win–win" strategies and tactics, rev edn. Crisp Publications, Menlo Park

 Further Reading

Eunson B 1994 Negotiation skills. John Wiley, Brisbane
Gibbs G, Habeshaw S, Habeshaw T 1986
    53 interesting ways to assess your students.
    Technical and Educational Services, Avon
Windschuttle K, Elliott E 1994 Writing, researching, communicating: communication skills for the information age, 2nd edn. McGraw-Hill, New York, pp. 393–400

10

Using experts

For any therapist new to research it is strongly advised that contributions be sought from a supervisor or mentor with research experience. If the research is part of a professional qualification this supervision will generally be provided by an academic from the institution awarding that qualification. In some situations a person outside the institution (e.g. a clinician, or someone from another discipline) may be involved as either the primary supervisor or as an associate supervisor.

The advice of other experts also may be required during various stages of the research process. These may include persons with expertise in research project management, research design and analysis, research methods, a specific clinical area or another discipline, equipment design and maintenance or computer programming. The manner in which the therapist interacts with these experts will have a bearing on the type of advice received and also the subsequent reputation of the therapist and the institution in which they are working. This chapter focuses mainly on the relationship between the researching therapist and a supervisor. Some suggestions are also provided on how to seek and use the advice of other experts.

Some aspects of the supervisory process are related to the role of the therapist as research student. To avoid confusion between this role and the role of another therapist as a supervisor, the term 'research student' will be used when referring to the novice researcher.

THE RESEARCH STUDENT–SUPERVISOR RELATIONSHIP

Collaborative research between a research student and a supervisor requires a substantial commitment of time and energy from both parties, not only to the project but also to developing a relationship which ensures the success of that project. The type of relationship that develops between the research student and the supervisor is affected by a number of factors, but most importantly by the personalities of the two parties, their communication skills, their respective learning and teaching styles, and by the model of supervision adopted. Three models have been identified which characterize the research student–supervisor relationship.

In the apprentice model (Moses 1985) the research student works with and for an experienced researcher (the supervisor) with the intention of 'learning the research trade'. At the end of the process the student is deemed sufficiently skilled to conduct research independently and to pass on their skills to others. This model is common in the natural and applied sciences. One concern with the apprentice model is the assumption that the supervisor is omniscient, and the locus of control is generally with the supervisor.

The coming of age model (Moses 1985) is encountered more frequently in the humanities and social sciences. In this model, after completing a prerequisite course of study (generally the undergraduate degree), the research student is deemed to have come of age and is bestowed the new freedoms of independent inquiry and undirected study. The supervisor takes on the role of 'parent', staying in the background to provide advice and counsel when the inevitable problems and setbacks occur. With this model there is the potential for the research student to be left floundering, which can be costly in terms of time and self-confidence. In this situation the student may perceive that the locus of control is with the supervisor.

The third and preferred model of supervision, the collegial model (Zuber-Skerritt 1992), considers the student and the supervisor to be engaged in a joint endeavour. As an adult learner, the research student is empowered with a degree of autonomy and is accepted into the research community. In the collegial model there is a degree of equity and mutual responsibility, and therefore control is shared between the supervisor and the student.

The type of model that is used will affect the functions and responsibilities of both the research student and the supervisor, and provides the framework within which they will operate. An important consideration is the locus of control or power that each of these models promotes, as this will have an influence on the selection process (i.e. matching of student and supervisor) and how the research topic is determined.

The model that will predominate in the research student–supervisor relationship should be discussed early, as conflicts between learning style and supervision style are a common reason for failure to develop a productive relationship (Moses 1985). As with any relationship the key is good communication. Openness and honesty are imperative when discussing progress and problems, as well as resolving disagreements on points regarding methods, analysis and interpretation.

Finally, the relationship between research student and supervisor should not be considered static, but rather its character should change over time (Connell 1985). As the relationship develops over the duration of the project it will become more equal, with the supervisor acting more as mentor than master, and both sharing the roles of teacher and learner.

One way of formalizing the research student–supervisor relationship is through a flexibly structured learning contract. Learning contracts have been used extensively in education, business and field-based practice as a method of minimizing conflict and promoting more productive relationships (Knowles 1986, Stephenson & Laycock, 1993). The contract is a document, developed collaboratively by the student and the supervisor, which specifies what skills the research student will develop, the methods by which they will be attained and the timeframe in which to achieve them, and identifies the methods of evaluation which will be directed toward the achievement of the research product (thesis, report, journal article). The role of the supervisor in assisting the research student to achieve these skills is also part of the agreement. The research student–supervisor contract is an agreement between the parties which promotes communication and clarification of the relationship at the outset, but which allows for some flexibility and individuality within the research process.

ROLE OF THE RESEARCH STUDENT

Conducting a research project can be a very different experience from other student or work experiences. As described in the previous section, one of the main features of the research experience is that the student will generally be guided throughout the process by a mentor or supervisor. Depending on the type of supervisory model used and the experience of the supervisor, the research student may be expected to fulfil certain roles and responsibilities. The following section outlines the types of activities which are generally considered to be the responsibility of the research student.

As there are generally significant financial and personal commitments associated with undertaking a research project the research student needs to accept responsibility for planning and executing the project within the timeframe allotted for the course or degree. In order to do this, the research student must set short- and long-term goals, in conjunction with the supervisor, and work *diligently* towards achieving these goals. Depending on the research student's previous experience, additional skills or knowledge may need to be acquired by undertaking coursework, independent study or other activities.

To ensure that the short-term goals are met in the appropriate timeframe the research student should meet regularly with the supervisor. In some situations this may require the student to take the initiative to arrange a meeting. It is their responsibility to plan and prepare for meetings and to document the proceedings (see Chapter 11, p. 74). During meetings the student should

report honestly on their progress and initiate discussion with the supervisor when a problem is encountered, demonstrating efforts to resolve the problem independently by offering options or potential solutions. It is also the student's responsibility to advise the supervisor as soon as possible of any problems (personal, academic, financial) which are impeding or may impede progress.

With regard to any written work presented to the supervisor it is the research student's responsibility to produce legible and readable material. As a matter of courtesy some effort should be spent proofreading, spell-checking and formatting written work before submitting it (see Chapter 14, p. 107). It is also in the student's best interest to seek advice and comments on their work from other research colleagues.

Finally, a significant part of the research student's role is as a member of the research community. As such, the research student should take responsibility to:

- Become a well-informed, active participant in the process of obtaining a research-based degree (be familiar with course requirements or institution policies and requirements for higher degrees)
- Ensure that all the administrative requirements of the institution (enrolment, annual reports, etc.) are met each semester
- Be familiar with and follow the institution's code of conduct for the responsible and ethical practice of research.

To be an active member of the intellectual and research community the research student should seek to participate in activities and opportunities offered by the institution. This may include attending and/or participating in seminars, meetings, courses and conferences.

As the student progresses through the project they should aim to demonstrate an increasing independence in performing the research activities. The level of independence should be commensurate with the level of the research project. Above all, the research student should generate and display enthusiasm and commitment to the project.

ROLE OF THE SUPERVISOR

As the research student–supervisor relationship is a partnership, the supervisor also has certain responsibilities. A number of these overlap with those of the research student, and in these cases the role of the supervisor is to guide the student and to encourage the development of independence.

Initially one of the roles of the supervisor is to discuss the choice of research topic and the nature of the project that will be undertaken. The supervisor should also outline the expected standard of research and any other expectations they have of the student. Once these issues have been covered, it is the role of the supervisor to assist the research student in planning the research programme and to provide ongoing support as the project progresses. To monitor the progress of the project a schedule of meetings should be set, with the frequency and duration determined in consultation with the student.

During the course of the research project the main role of the supervisor is to monitor progress in relation to the specified timeframe. The supervisor may need to help the research student find or maintain the appropriate focus (narrow/broad, specific area) so that the goals can be met and the project can be finished on time. The supervisor should be familiar with the institution's regulations and requirements, and specifically they should be familiar with the procedures related to the submission of the final report or thesis.

With regard to written work, the supervisor has a responsibility to the research student to provide written feedback and to participate in discussion of the work with the student. Feedback should be provided within an appropriate timeframe.

Finally, it is also the responsibility of the supervisor to generate and display enthusiasm and commitment to the research project.

ISSUES FOR DISCUSSION WITH A PROSPECTIVE/NEW SUPERVISOR

Depending on the supervisory model desired, the research student may seek a supervisor with a research idea in mind or they may choose to work with a specific supervisor based on that supervisor's area of research interest. There are a number of questions that the research student should discuss with prospective supervisors:

- Is the project feasible; are adequate resources available?
- Can the project be completed within the suggested timeframe?
- Does the topic have appropriate scope for the level of the project?
- Does the supervisor have knowledge of the area of interest?
- Do the research student's background and skills fit the topic of interest?
- How well defined is the topic? will the research student need to read widely in order to narrow down the research question?
- Does the research student need to improve their knowledge in specific areas? If so, are there courses available or will it require primarily independent study?
- What facilities and resources are available to the research student (desk or study space, computer facilities, photocopying, interlibrary loan fees, funding/research grants, opportunities for work (tutoring))?
- What expectations does the institution have of the research student?

DEVELOPING A RESEARCH STUDENT–SUPERVISOR CONTRACT

If the research student and supervisor agree to collaborate on a project, discussions may lead to the development of a contract. The research student is generally responsible for writing up such a contract, based on discussions with the supervisor. The contract should be a written account of the issues discussed and agreed to, and each party should be provided with a signed copy.

The issues which may be addressed in the contract have been grouped under three headings: managing the relationship, selecting the project and managing the project.

Managing the relationship

- Discussions regarding preferred learning and supervisory styles
- Work style of the prospective research student
- Access to the supervisor outside scheduled meeting times
- The type and amount of supervision the research student needs/desires and what the supervisor is able to provide
- The procedures that will be used for monitoring the supervision process and the problem-solving strategies which may be employed if difficulties develop between supervisor and student
- Any relevant personal circumstances that affect the supervision or completion of the project.

Selecting the project

- The process of selecting the research topic: joint or unilateral
- The scope of the proposed project in terms of amount of work that will be required, and type, structure and length of the final report or thesis
- Expected timeframe of the project (completion date that considers the course or degree requirement, scholarship requirements and personal commitments)
- Role of associate supervisors
- Access to institutional resources and equipment; standard procedures and protocols
- Issues related to authorship.

Managing the project

- Frequency, duration and content of meetings; who is responsible for initiating meetings; who is responsible for managing the meetings; protocol to be followed when one party is unable to attend
- Expected frequency and content of progress reports
- Expectations regarding feedback: how much, how often, in what form, in what timeframe?

- Procedures for managing problems when the supervisor is absent
- Processes for determining and ensuring an equitable distribution of workload in a multiple-student project.

JOINT SUPERVISION

The interdisciplinary nature of a research topic may require that more than one main supervisor is involved with the project (Phillips & Pugh 1990). Having more than one supervisor modifies the typical relationship that develops between research student and supervisor, and requires some additional effort from all parties to ensure that the learning process is fostered and that the project is successful. When discussing the student–supervisor contract special attention should be paid to defining the specific roles each supervisor will take in terms of theoretical or technical advice and the administrative responsibilities associated with research student progress and the final written document. Where possible, joint meetings should be organized regularly so that both supervisors are aware of the suggestions that are given to the student. This will reduce confusion and avert some of the potential conflict a research student may experience. If joint meetings cannot be arranged, then an accurate record of what occurs in separate meetings should be kept and promptly distributed to both supervisors, to keep them informed of progress and suggestions. If advice received from the supervisors is conflicting it is important to first determine whether it is a major or a minor conflict: if it is only minor the research student will generally benefit from following both suggestions, even though it might require a little more work. If a major conflict in advice occurs the problem is probably best addressed in a joint meeting.

USING AN EXPERT IN RESEARCH DESIGN AND ANALYSIS

Regardless of the type of research being conducted, it is always advisable to seek the advice of an expert in research design and analysis, such as a statistician, epidemiologist or conceptual analyst. Such advice may be required at several stages during the research project, generally during the development of the proposal and later, once the data have been collected and are ready for analysis.

Unfortunately, many researchers fail to seek such expert advice during the development of the research proposal, yet this is probably the most crucial time for their input. Appropriate advice early in the project will ensure that the chosen design is suitable and that the resultant data will adequately address the research question.

During the development of the proposal the expert in research design and analysis may assist the student with advice on the following:

- Selection of a research design (e.g. qualitative or quantitative)
- Formulation of any hypotheses or guiding questions
- Descriptions of the characteristics of the data produced by the proposed measures and any assumptions that may be required about the distribution of the data
- Selection of the statistical model to be applied to test any hypotheses
- Calculations of sample size and power
- Selection of an appropriate qualitative analysis approach
- The design of pilot studies that may be needed to determine effect size or the reliability of measures.

In some cases the supervisor is chosen specifically for their expertise in a particular research design or analysis. In other situations the supervisor is chosen for their expertise in the area being studied, and the research student and supervisor together may choose to seek the advice of an expert in statistics and research design. In this situation the expert may require some background information and detailed descriptions of the methods to be used. Providing a copy of the Introduction, Literature Review and Methods sections of the research proposal prior to the meeting may be useful. In addition, the research student must be able to articulate to the expert the research question and any related hypotheses or guiding questions which may have been developed to answer it. The research student must also be prepared to provide information about the data which will be collected. The following are some examples of the types of questions the research expert may ask:

- What type of data will be collected?
- How many independent groups will be tested?
- Will subjects be tested on more than one occasion?
- What is the proposed sample size?
- Is the intention to describe the data or to make inferences about the population?
- Is there a convention in the literature about how the results from research in the specific area of study are analysed or presented?

USING OTHER EXPERTS

Depending on the nature of the project, the research student may need to consult other experts such as technicians, computer programmers, librarians and lay people. In all situations where a research student requires the assistance of an expert, good communications skills are the key to a successful interaction. The research student should make every effort to provide the individual with sufficient background information so that they may understand the nature of the request. The request should then be posed using clear and concise language.

The advice of a supervisor and other relevant experts will be important to the success of the research project. The researching therapist should use these resources wisely.

REFERENCES

Connell R 1985 How to supervise a PhD. Vestes 2: 38–41
Knowles M 1986 Using learning contracts. Jossey-Bass, San Francisco
Moses I 1985 Supervising postgraduates. Higher Education Research and Development Society of Australasia, Kensington, NSW

Phillips E, Pugh D 1990 How to get a PhD. Open University Press, Philadelphia

Zuber-Skerritt 1992 Starting research: supervision and training. Tertiary Education Institute, Brisbane

 Further Reading

Curtin University of Technology 1994 Handbook of guidelines and regulations for higher degrees by research. Curtin University of Technology, Perth

Stephenson J, Laycock M 1993 Using learning contracts in higher education. Kogan Page, London

University of Sydney 1994 Responsibilities of the candidate. In: Postgraduate studies handbook. University of Sydney, Sydney

Using time wisely

Time is one of the researcher's most valuable resources. Unfortunately, only one rule holds true with regard to time: it can neither be saved nor substituted, it can only be spent. The key to success, therefore, is the ability to spend or use one's time wisely.

Often there will be a specific timeframe within which a research project must be completed (particularly if it is conducted as part of a course or degree). The consequence of this is that the time available must be managed well, so that the project finishes on time with all of the goals having been met. The key concept here is that of management. Using one's time wisely requires attentiveness and effort on an ongoing basis. The aim of this chapter is to highlight some time management strategies that may be used by the researching therapist.

THE TIME MANAGEMENT PROCESS

Using time wisely is not a matter of working longer or working harder; effective time management is the result of planning so that the time available is used productively. Planning also provides a framework for decision making, whether the decisions are made in advance or in the midst of a crisis. Planning does, however, require the investment of some time.

The first step in developing a time management plan involves identifying goals. This includes both broad or long-term goals and more specific short-term goals, which can then be divided into weekly or daily objectives. Once these have been identified, priorities can be set and a daily action plan developed.

Establishing the goals and objectives for a research project is an important step in the planning process and requires considerable thought. Whereas the major targets required to complete a research project are generally more obvious (write a research proposal, select a sample, collect the necessary data, analyse the data and write up the report), the steps which must be followed to reach those targets are often less obvious, particularly to the novice researcher. Thus, the researching therapist should call on the experience of others in the research community, including the supervisor(s) and other students/therapists.

In developing the list of goals and objectives consideration must also be given to any obstacles that might be encountered and strategies that may be needed to overcome them or minimize their effects. For the novice researcher the main obstacles are lack of experience and skills. Consequently, the plan will need to include sufficient time and resources for these to be developed. Other obstacles might include the availability of participants and the need to share research equipment or space.

Before consideration is given to the daily action list and other time management tools two important concepts must be examined. The first involves breaking the day into blocks, according to patterns of personal energy and creativity and the potential influence of external time constraints. The second involves assessing the characteristics of individual tasks so that they can be prioritized and allocated to the appropriate times of the day.

Prime time

Most people find that their energy varies during the day and that there are certain times when they are more productive. For time to be used most effectively, it is important to determine how these energy levels vary through a typical day. This can be done by creating a graph similar to the one in Figure 11.1. The period of maximum energy and concentration is called 'prime time'.

Three verbs should be applied to prime time: respect, protect and direct (Clark & Clark 1994). As this period has been identified as the time when energy and concentration is highest, this time must be respected and the available energy be applied diligently. Protecting prime time gen-

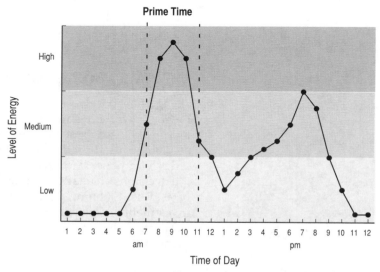

Figure 11.1 A plot of variations in perceived energy level throughout a typical day, with the prime time period identified

erally means blocking off this period each day and working to ensure that unimportant activities do not creep in. Having done this, the available energy should be directed to the task which has been set as the main priority for that day. By consciously planning to perform key activities during prime time and matching other tasks to energy levels during the rest of the day, productivity can be improved.

Determining task priorities

Characteristics which should be considered when prioritizing tasks include the time required to complete the task, the degree of mental energy required, urgency and locus of control. Careful planning and consideration of these will enable a greater number of tasks to be fitted into the day.

Some consideration needs to be given to the projected duration of each task. If the task is unfamiliar it may be difficult to estimate how much time is required. The danger in this situation is to underestimate, and it seems that research activities often take two to three times as long as might appear necessary at first glance.

The researcher should aim to place each task into one of three categories, according to the time required to complete it. The first category will contain tasks which take 1–4 hours to complete; the second will consist of tasks which take more than 10 minutes but less than an hour to finish; and the last category is for quick tasks which take less than 10 minutes. Very large tasks, i.e. greater than 4 hours' duration, should be broken down into subtasks until the subtasks can be assigned to one of the three categories. An example of a very large task would be writing the Literature Review: this can be broken down by dividing the review into major subheadings and further dividing it by listing the main points to be covered in each section. The advantage of keeping the number of categories to three, with a maximum duration of 4 hours, is that the tasks can be more readily scheduled into the day, and as a greater number of tasks can actually be completed the researcher will gain a sense of achievement at the end of each day.

The second characteristic to consider is the mental energy each task requires. Some research activities require high levels of creativity or concentration (e.g. writing), whereas others can be considered more menial (e.g. maintaining the reference database and filing articles). Tasks which require the greatest mental energy should be scheduled for prime time.

Probably the most obvious characteristic which affects task priority is urgency. Again three categories may be established. Category A activities are those that have the highest urgency (i.e. tasks which, if not completed that day, will have a catastrophic outcome). Category B activities are those to which a deadline for completion can be assigned. Category C activities are those tasks or activities that would be nice to do but do not necessarily have a deadline. Naturally, category A activities should be placed high on the priority list: these are the only types of activities that should be allowed to creep unscheduled into prime time. The majority of tasks will fall into category B, and with good planning and diligence they should not become category A.

The last task characteristic to consider is the locus of control (i.e. internal or external). An internal locus of control is where the researcher has control over when a task can be done. An external locus of control involves tasks whose scheduling is controlled by someone else, tasks which require others to be present (e.g. subjects) or tasks which can only be done at certain times of the day.

A number of other task characteristics can be identified which do not necessarily affect priority but may be important for efficiency. These can be assessed by asking the following questions:

- Can the task be delegated to someone else?
- Will the same or a similar task need to be performed in the future?
- Can the task be standardized or automated?

If the last two questions produce an affirmative response, the researcher should consider devoting additional time to these tasks in the short term so that time can be saved in the long term. Spending time learning how to use a computer program (e.g. a wordprocessor or statistics program) is an example of this type of task. Some research activities (such as data reduction) can be automated using computers or other equipment, significantly improving efficiency.

Hazard 11.1

Unfamiliar tasks often take longer to complete than expected

STRATEGIES FOR TIME MANAGEMENT

Possibly the most important strategy for time management is including time (ideally 10–15 minutes) in each day to plan. Planning may occur at the beginning or at the end of the day; however, there are a number of advantages to planning at the end of the day. Planning in advance gives the researcher a head start when they arrive at their workstation, starting each day or session with a sense of direction. Based on the current day's activities, any tasks which have not been completed can be reassessed and the priority changed if necessary. Finally, spending the last 15 minutes of the day planning contributes to a sense of closure, providing the researcher with a sense of accomplishment.

The daily action list

Regardless of the time of day which is devoted to planning, the primary goal of the planning time is to develop the daily action list (i.e. the list of all tasks that need to be accomplished). Tasks should be grouped into categories based on size, and within each category the list should be prioritized according to urgency. Having a daily action list will prevent time being wasted, as it will be immediately obvious what needs to be done and suitable tasks can be chosen to fill in any gaps that develop in the schedule.

Larger tasks and tasks with an external locus of control should be scheduled using an appointment calendar. When preparing an appointment calendar, time should be blocked off each day for prime time and planning, and other appoint-

ments and meetings should be scheduled around these blocks.

It is important to be realistic when developing the daily action list and appointment calendar as there is often the temptation to include more tasks in the list than can actually be completed in the time. This will not increase productivity, but will certainly decrease motivation when the end of the day is reached before the end of the list.

To facilitate the development of the daily action list a master list of activities should be prepared. This is essentially the list of objectives which were determined when considering the goals for the research project (some objectives may need to be broken down to create more manageable tasks). Any additional tasks which arise or come to mind during the day should be placed on the master list immediately. During the daily planning period selected tasks are transferred from the master list to the daily action list for the next day. Tasks from the previous day which have not been completed can either be transferred to the next day's action list or returned to the master list.

Research meetings

Meetings with supervisors and colleagues are one of the activities that should be scheduled regularly to keep the project moving purposefully towards completion (Fanning 1990). Planning for such meetings, however short or seemingly informal, is imperative. Even if the meeting is informal an agenda should be set which outlines the topics to be covered. These can be classified into three categories: information for exchange only, items which require discussion, and items which require a decision. To ensure that the most important topics are covered the list should be assessed and the meeting should begin with those of greatest priority. The natural flow of the meeting may see the discussion move from one category to the other, but having an agenda will ensure that the meeting time is used wisely and that important topics are not missed.

A second aspect of planning a research meeting is documentation (Fig. 11.2). Once an agenda has been set, all parties attending the meeting

Research Meeting Agenda

Date: Sept 2, 1997

Attendees: Student 1, Student 2, Student 3, Student 4, Supervisor A and Supervisor B

Topic	Points discussed	Decisions made or follow up required
1. Modifications to the computer literacy and anxiety questionnaire	• Changes to items 2, 3, 5, 14 and 22 to suit sample • Items 32 to 55 cannot be changed as this will affect the validity and reliability	• Additional items added to clarify problems with item 20 • Students 1 and 2 to modify questionnaire layout • Supervisor A to provide electronic copy of existing questionnaire
2. Funding for administration of questionnaire	• Supervisor B spoke to course coordinator, some funding is available	• Once costs have been estimated Supervisor B will request funds from course coordinator
3. Additional instrument to measure state and trait anxiety	• Instrument would need to be short	• Supervisor A to contact Psychology Tests librarian
4. First draft of Literature Review	• Due to other assignments being due the draft was not completed	• Students to make available to Supervisors A and B before the end of the week
5. Methods		• First draft to be ready for next meeting

etc.

Figure 11.2 An example of a research meeting agenda and documentation of the discussion related to each topic on the agenda

should be given a copy. This gives each individual the opportunity to be prepared. If there is any material that must be read by one or more of the parties (e.g. the supervisor), this should also be provided well in advance of the meeting date. During the meeting the researcher should document which topics have been covered, the major points discussed, and any decision or action stemming from the discussion. Annotation can

be directly on the agenda if sufficient writing space has been allocated.

For the research meeting to be successful the time of the other individuals participating in the meeting must be respected. For this reason, every effort should be made to start and finish the meeting on time, and discussions should be directed to the topic at hand. Topics of lesser importance or not related to the research project should only be discussed after the agenda items have been dealt with.

DEALING WITH THINGS THAT INTERFERE WITH TIME MANAGEMENT

There are three things which may arise that, despite one's best efforts at time management, can be disruptive. These are interruptions, crises and procrastination.

Managing interruptions

Even the best-planned schedule is not immune to interruptions. Three types of interruptions are common: drop-in visitors, interruptions by colleagues and telephone calls. Managing these interruptions generally requires assertiveness skills. The following suggestions may be useful:

- Say 'No' if asked to perform extra tasks. Protect the research priorities and decline tactfully but firmly requests that do not contribute to the achievement of specific research goals.
- Meet visitors outside the office, or greet them by standing up: remaining seated acts as an open invitation for someone to pull up a chair and stay.
- Set a time limit at the beginning of the conversation (this applies to telephone and in-person interruptions). For example, 'I only have 10 minutes to talk right now, is that enough time or should we schedule a meeting (can I call you back) later?'
- Develop techniques for closing conversations: these can be verbal or non-verbal (glancing at a watch, clock or diary; clearing the desktop, standing up).
- During prime time use an answering machine to screen telephone calls that can be returned during low energy periods.
- If there is a door to the office close it, particularly during prime time.
- If the research space is shared with others, consider setting a specific quiet time.

Managing crises

All good plans include a contingency plan for when something unexpected occurs. In research crises are generally related to one of the following: problems with research equipment or computers; conflicts with the supervisor or colleagues; personal matters; and other factors which result in failure to meet deadlines. The best way to control a crisis is to avoid it. This may be accomplished by trying to anticipate problems and implementing solutions before the problem becomes a crisis. Most people will generally be able to handle a single crisis: the real problem occurs when two or more crises develop concurrently, as they have a multiplicative rather than additive effect. However, some crises can neither be avoided nor anticipated. The best way to manage any crisis is to stand back and attempt to consider the problem from a non-emotive viewpoint. Priorities can then be re-evaluated and non-essential activities cancelled or rescheduled. Once the priority task has been determined the researcher's energy should be focused on completing that task before moving on to the next (when pressured, people often try to do several things at once, reducing efficiency and contributing to an increased sense of pressure). In times of crisis the time management strategies discussed in this chapter become even more valuable, and some effort should be directed towards planning, prioritizing, controlling interruptions and avoiding procrastination. When the crisis has been resolved the researching therapist should take some time to evaluate the precursors to the crisis, so that similar problems may be identified and further crises prevented.

Conquering procrastination

Procrastination is probably the greatest threat to successful completion of the research project. Psychologists have identified several reasons why people procrastinate, including fear of failure, fear of success, and fear of surrendering control.

The most important tool for conquering a tendency to procrastinate is the daily action list, as it gives a clear indication of what needs to be accomplished. Once the task that must be done has been identified, the best way to begin is to physically put oneself in front of it. This may involve getting the necessary files out and placing them on the desk, or it may involve physically moving to another location (e.g. the library, laboratory or computer room).

In most cases this initial action will be sufficient to overcome the urge to do nothing; if not, it is possible that the task is perceived as being either unpleasant or difficult. Unfortunately, many tasks associated with research can at times be considered unpleasant or difficult. The best way to overcome this continued hesitation is to commit a specified time (e.g. 10 minutes) to work earnestly on the task. At the end of the specified time the commitment to continuing to work on the task can be re-evaluated. Generally, once the initial problem with inertia is overcome most tasks become engaging.

PROJECT TIMELINES

An important aspect of time management with respect to meeting research deadlines is developing and using a project timeline.

A number of project mapping approaches have been developed in order to help plan and monitor progress. Common graphical representations are the PERT chart, the critical path method and the Gantt chart. The method described here combines the strengths of each of these and gives some examples of how they may be used to manage a research project.

A common approach to planning is to consider the current status of a project and the end product or goal and then to outline the steps (objectives) which are necessary to reach that goal. Once the steps have been identified, the length of time required to complete each step may be determined and the projected completion date calculated by adding up the total time required to complete all steps. This approach uses 'forward' thinking.

An alternate approach is to use 'backward' thinking. This method begins with the completed product (and target completion date) and then considers which tasks or activities must be fin-

ished before the final product can be put together. This process is repeated, working backwards to identify all tasks which must be completed before work can begin on the next task in the sequence. Planning 'backwards' requires a bit more thought and concentration, and may help to identify activities that are necessary to the process but which might otherwise be missed.

Using either backward or forward thinking, each component of the research project can be described by listing all of the tasks required to complete it. The relationships between the components can then be considered. When evaluating each of the tasks in a component and the relationship between components, it becomes apparent that some tasks must be completed before others begin, whereas other tasks can be done at any time. Tasks that are dependent on others can be linked to create a critical path. Outlining the critical path helps to establish priorities when creating the daily action list.

Having established a list of all of the steps that need to be completed in the research project and identifying which activities are on the critical path, the timeframes for each task and component can be established. All of these components can be brought together and represented graphically using a Gantt-style chart.

This is similar to a (horizontal) bar chart, in that the x axis represents time, whereas the y axis categorizes the different tasks required to complete the project. The relative length of each task is shown by the length of the bar. Groups of subtasks and important milestones are identified using brackets and other symbols (Fig. 11.3). A vertical line corresponding to the current date helps to identify daily priorities and demonstrates concurrent tasks.

Gantt charts have many advantages, including the ability to show how activities are interrelated and to identify the critical path; help identify trouble spots or potential crises; and manage delays, communicate progress and planned activities with others (e.g. supervisors and colleagues). Gantt-style charts are often included in the research proposal to indicate the projected timelines for the research study.

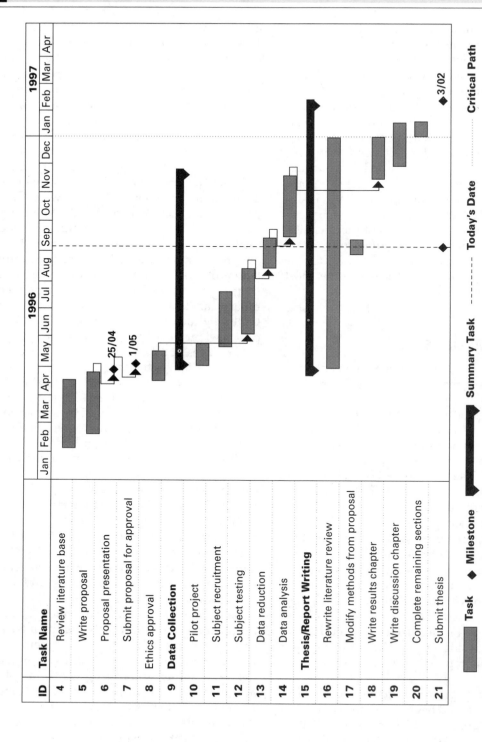

Figure 11.3   An example of a Gantt-style project chart illustrating the main components of the project, their subtasks and milestones and the timelines associated with each of these. The critical path for specific components of the project is also identified

This chapter has considered a number of time management strategies to help the researching therapist to identify and prioritize the research tasks and to match them to variations in daily mental and physical energy, so that the goals of the research project can be met within the desired timeframe.

REFERENCES

Clark J, Clark S 1994 How to make the most of your workday. Career Press, Hawthorne, NJ
Fanning T 1990 Get it all done and still be human: a personal time management workshop. Kali House, Menlo Park, CA

Further Reading

Garratt S 1985 Manage your time. Fontana/Collins, London
Gleeson K 1994 The personal efficiency program: how to get organized to do more work in less time. Wiley, New York

Managing data and controlling quality

Often, insufficient thought and effort is devoted to the task of implementing the research project. Some researchers find the data collection and data entry phases less intellectually stimulating than designing the study and interpreting the results. If adequate attention is not paid during the data collection and entry phases, errors may be introduced into the data. These errors may be obvious (e.g. missing data) or hidden (e.g. systematic errors in measurement), but in either case the problem is difficult to resolve after the event and impacts upon the validity and trustworthiness of the findings and the conclusions that can be drawn from the study (Hulley & Cummings 1988). Vigilance and a structured approach to the collection and management of data will ensure that quality data are used for analysis and interpretation. This chapter provides suggestions for monitoring the quality of data. Guidelines are provided for the development of a project file and are followed by recommendations regarding the design of data collection forms and an outline of the processes used to monitor data quality. The importance of pilot studies and a well rehearsed approach to data collection is also highlighted.

THE PROJECT FILE

The project file includes specific details on how to proceed with the various steps required to implement the study: pilot studies, subject/participant recruitment, measurement or data collection procedures, data reduction and data analysis. Having specific written instructions for each of these steps will reduce both random variation and systematic errors which may be introduced into the data. Constructing and maintaining a project file also facilitates writing up the project by ensuring that relevant details are recorded along the way.

Depending on the scope of the project the project file may be extremely comprehensive, including administrative details necessary to organize and implement a large-scale study or multicentre trial, or less expansive in the case of a smaller study involving only one researcher. The contents of a project file can be grouped into three main categories, relating to the management of subjects, data and the project overall. As the size of the file increases it may be useful to partition these sections and to include a table of contents to facilitate quick access to the information.

As an introduction to the file it is useful to write a brief summary of the study, including its purpose and the perceived benefits to the subjects, the community or the profession. This can be used as an introduction to potential subjects when recruiting by telephone, and may also form the basis of a response to inquiries about the study. Inquiries may be made by representatives of the media or by others seeking information about the project in order to promote the institution or profession (e.g. for institutional annual reports, quality assessment committees, professional newsletters) or to evaluate the project's progress (e.g. student progress reports, interim reports to granting agencies).

Subject management

This section includes details related to subject/participant recruitment and communication with subjects throughout the study.

With regard to subject recruitment, an outline of the various strategies to be used should be included. A record of information pamphlets or posters, press releases and newspaper articles or advertisements should be kept in case a further recruiting drive is needed to meet the desired sample size. The researcher may choose to keep track of details such as the current rate of recruitment in relation to the rate necessary to meet the proposed sample size in the allotted time, and the relative success of different strategies (this may be useful for future studies). If stratified sampling techniques are used it is also important to keep a running total of subjects from each stratum.

To assist with the process of subject recruitment the researcher may choose to design a form similar to the one in Appendix C. This is particularly useful for telephone recruiting, as it ensures that all the relevant questions are asked of each respondent to determine their suitability for inclusion in the study. A detailed set of guidelines for inclusion and exclusion should also be recorded in the project file, and should be kept close at hand so that appropriate and consistent decisions can be made. The subject recruitment and follow-up form also serves as a record of the number of respondents which were excluded or withdrawn from the study, and the reasons why. This information will have implications for the generalizability of the findings and should be summarized in the final research report. Depending on the specificity of the recruiting techniques applied a large proportion of the respondents may be deemed unsuitable; consequently, this approach may be a useful way of managing this information even if the target sample size is relatively small.

In managing participants in the study it may be necessary to keep track of follow-up visits. Both the timing and content of the visits should be clearly outlined in the project file, and the procedures for following non-responders should be described. If subjects are to be assigned to groups the method (e.g. random assignment) should be described and the number of subjects assigned to each group should be recorded as a running total. The project file should also contain the original copy of all material that needs to be sent or given to subjects. This may include appointment cards, parking stickers, maps or instructions for locating the testing facility, and instructions regarding activities prior to or between testing sessions.

As the study progresses there may be other

types of correspondence with subjects, which may be included in the project file or filed elsewhere.

Data management

The data management portion of the project file organizes and outlines the specific procedures required to collect the necessary data. It also contains a study log in which activities related to data collection are recorded.

Data may be collected in a variety of ways depending on the type of research being performed. In quantitative studies data may be collected by writing results directly on a form or questionnaire, or be recorded as output from some measurement or recording device. For qualitative studies data may be collected by questionnaire or from interviews, participant observation, examination of written documents or evaluation of various media (e.g. film, art).

Guidelines for developing data collection forms are outlined on page 84 and the processes used to monitor data quality are described on page 86.

After the necessary forms (e.g. data collection and consent forms) or questionnaires have been developed the original copy should be kept in the project file. Keeping all the forms in one place guarantees quick and easy access for photocopying. Detailed instructions for filling in data forms and transposing data into a data file should also be included. Similarly, descriptions of all coding conventions and other data reduction procedures should be included in the project file.

To guide the collection of data (primarily quantitative data) each variable should be operationally defined: this definition should include specific details of how the measurement is to be performed or obtained (see Chapter 5 for a description of operational definitions). In qualitative research operational notes may be used to guide the interview or data collection process. During the study the researcher should refer back to these definitions to ensure that a consistent approach is maintained throughout the data collection period. Even measurements that are

difficult to make at first can become easy with repetition, and this may lead to sloppy practices. Simple measures are particularly prone to quality degradation for this reason.

If the study uses an experimental or quasi-experimental design, in which an intervention is to be applied to a subject group(s), a detailed description of the intervention should be developed and included in the project file to ensure that the intervention is applied consistently to each member of the group.

If several procedures or measures are to be applied to each subject it is useful to place a checklist on the front of a file or folder for each subject. It will be immediately apparent from a quick glance at this list which procedures have or have not been completed, thereby helping to prevent missing data.

For projects involving equipment the data management section of the project file should include a list of all the equipment that will be needed. This is particularly important if the researcher does not have access to a designated area where equipment can be set up and left. The use of a checklist and the allocation of preparation time will ensure that valuable time with a subject is not wasted searching for or setting up equipment. If complex equipment set-ups are required (e.g. camera and equipment set up for movement analysis) these should also be described or illustrated in a diagram so that day-to-day variability is reduced (see Appendix D for examples of combined equipment checklist and set-up instructions).

In developing the equipment list it is also useful to record the specific details of all instruments to be used, including the full name of all major devices/programs and the manufacturer or copyright holder's name and address (e.g. KinCom 500H, Chattanooga Group Inc., Hixson, Tennessee, USA). This information is often required when reporting the methods in journal articles or theses, and having it to hand can save time later.

Instruments and equipment used for research often need to be calibrated to ensure that the output corresponds to the input and that the variability is minimal across the range of values to be collected. The procedures for and frequency of calibration should be outlined in the project file, and a record of calibration dates and values kept.

If complex computer file-naming procedures are used (either created manually by the researcher or automatically by the computer software) these should be outlined: what appears obvious one day can seem like hieroglyphics with the passing of time. For example, during a study of the ergonomics of combined lifting tasks a four-digit file name could be used to specify subject identification number, task type and frequency of lifting.

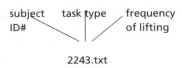

Example 12.1

Computer operating systems that accept file names longer than eight characters allow greater flexibility in file-naming procedures.

The second main element of the data management section of the procedures file is the study log. This is a simple record of the day-to-day activities associated with data collection. These include records of equipment calibration or maintenance, environmental conditions of the laboratory, dates when data files were backed up, any changes in protocol, and the occurrence of untoward events or problems and their solutions. The study log may also be used as a diary in which ideas or thoughts which arise during data collection, analysis or writing are recorded. These may act as triggers for additional lines of inquiry or discussion and may significantly improve the quality of the research. As these ideas often arise while performing other activities (e.g. measuring subjects) it is important that they are recorded as soon as possible, otherwise there is the risk that they may be forgotten. Putting thought into a more concrete form can also help the researcher to identify the merits or problems with a particular line of thinking.

Qualitative researchers often use a diary, sometimes referred to as a memo log, as an integral part of the research method. Memos are used as a record of the researcher's thoughts about the data or the research process. Diagrams can also be used to graphically represent relationships between concepts which may arise during the analysis of the data. Strauss and Corbin (1990) define several types of memos as they relate to the products of the coding process (code notes), the results of inductive or deductive thinking (theoretical notes) and ideas about the research process itself (operational notes). Although the actual technique used for producing the memos may vary (computer programs, colour-coded cards or notebooks), it is important that the contents are maintained in an orderly and systematic fashion which facilitates sorting, retrieval and cross-referencing. Each memo should be dated and classified (according to the above types) and include a reference to the trigger for the memo (i.e. the document or transcript being coded).

One final aspect of the data management process which must be considered is the archiving of data at the end of the project. Regardless of the type of data or the research paradigm used for collection, all institutions conducting research have a responsibility to the community to be able to provide details of any research conducted. This responsibility lasts for a specific time (generally 5–7 years) after the research is first reported. Some institutions may have specific guidelines or policies related to data retention: these should outline the types of data that must be archived and the format for the archive (hard copy or digital backup). Where feasible, the original primary data should be retained. This may, however, depend on the perishability of the data and the logistics of retaining them in their original form. Whether the primary data or the results of secondary data reduction or analysis are retained, the archived data should include sufficient detail to permit their authenticity to be established or to confirm the validity of the conclusions, and to permit re-examination in response to questions that may result from unintentional errors or misinterpretation.

Project management

Whether performed by a single researcher or by several, a research project requires management to ensure that it is completed on time and that the resultant product is of a high quality. These factors should not be left to chance but should be planned. Consequently, a section of the project file is devoted to the overall management of the project. This should include a detailed timeline with specific milestones and completion dates outlined (see Chapter 11, p. 77). If the project involves several individuals (or committees) each person's contribution to the project or responsibilities should be clearly outlined. Chapters 9 and 10 provide some suggestions for managing group processes and the student–supervisor relationship. One important suggestion is the use of a meeting log or diary, which summarizes what has been discussed at meetings and the actions required before the next meeting. This may be included in the project file.

All research projects require financial resources for equipment purchase / maintenance, consumables and personnel. Often some or all of these costs are absorbed by the institution (e.g. hospital, university), but other costs must be paid by the researcher or from research funds. Regardless of the source of funds, an initial budget and ongoing accounts should be maintained. It would be advisable to include these in this section of the project file.

Finally, project management includes the handling of correspondence, which may include letters of approval from ethics committees, letters to primary providers (referring physicians or therapists), progress reports (to supervisors, graduate committees or funding agencies), and communications with other sites in multicentre trials. Records of all communications should be maintained either in the project file or in a separate file.

DESIGNING THE DATA COLLECTION FORMS

Using the term broadly, data collection forms are forms on which the results of various measures, questions or observations are recorded. The following discussion focuses on data collection forms completed by the researcher, but the points raised may also be applied to the design of questionnaires in general. Regardless of the length or complexity of the form, it is important to spend time organizing and testing it to ensure that it will assist the data collection process rather than hinder it. The design of the form should also facilitate encoding and transposition of the data to a computer file. It follows, then, that some consideration needs to be given to the visual design of the form to make it easier for the subject or operator to complete it accurately. Although it may be advantageous to keep the information on one or only a few pages, it is important to provide sufficient space between items so that the form does not appear cluttered, and to provide adequate space to make the entries. If the form extends over more than one page, space for the subject number should be included on each page to ensure that the subject can be identified should the pages become separated.

When designing a form the same principles that guide the layout of a written document apply. Information about a particular topic or measure should be grouped together and distinguished by a descriptive heading. Variations in the left margin (indenting) also serve to organize the information and create the impression of a hierarchical order to the elements. These two visual cues and other techniques, such as the use of space, can be employed to create a form which is attractive and easy to use.

Good form design also considers that there should be a logical flow from one question or element to the next. For data collection forms the flow refers to the order in which the data will be written.

For questionnaires the flow refers to the path that the participant / operator takes from the first question to the final entry. In some cases this is simply linear; in other cases the path may branch, depending upon the answer to certain questions. For questionnaires that use branching questions the path should be made clear either by instructions (e.g. go to question 6) or by visual directors such as arrows.

5. *Have you ever used a computer to perform a statistical analysis?*

        [ ] Yes → Go to question 6

        [ ] No   → Go to question 9

Example 12.2

The order of questions depends somewhat on the purpose of the questionnaire. For some questionnaires there will be a logical flow, starting with general questions related to subject demographics (name, age, gender, etc.) and ending with more specific questions. At times the questions may be deliberately mixed to avoid leading the respondent along a theme, or so that questions which investigate the same or similar phenomena are not closely juxtaposed. In some cases, where sensitive issues are being investigated, the more challenging or sensitive questions may be left to the end so as to build up the subject's trust or confidence through the introductory questions.

As mentioned earlier, the visual structure of the form may involve changes in the vertical alignment of the left margin. An example of this is the organization of the options available to answer a closed-ended question. If the number of options is fewer than three they may be presented on a horizontal line; if more than three options are available they should be lined up vertically below the question (an exception to this would be a Likert scale, which generally contains five options and is presented horizontally). The list of options should be indented so that the questions remain distinct from the answers. Instructions to the subject or operator as to how they should indicate their choice should be clearly stated, and should specify whether more than one answer may be selected (e.g. Circle the number beside the sentence that best describes your feelings; place a tick in one of the boxes). The choices should be preceded by a number to be circled or by a box or brackets in which to place a tick ($\sqrt{}$) (see example 12.3).

Coding is an important component of form design as it transforms the answers into variables that can be used for analysis (Hulley & Cummings 1988). Precoded forms will signifi-

cantly improve the accuracy and efficiency of transferring the information to a data file. The answers to closed-ended questions can be pre-coded and the codes included on the form. Open-ended questions are generally coded after the interview or session, and space should be provided in the right-hand margin of the form for the code to be entered. Where possible, detailed procedures for coding open-ended questions should be developed prior to testing or as soon as possible during the data reduction process, to ensure consistent and reliable coding of responses.

Which leg would you use to kick a ball? (circle one number)

    1. left

    2. right

    3. either

Which leg would you use to kick a ball? (tick one)

    [ ] *left*

    [ ] *right*

    [ ] *either*

Example 12.3

The necessity for precoding is somewhat dependent on the type of analysis which will be performed and on the statistical package or analysis programs that may be used. If the statistical package does not support descriptive data categories (gender = male, female) then these must be converted to numeric values (gender: male = 1, female = 2). For simple coding these numbers can be included in the check box. To avoid errors, choices common to more than one test item should be coded the same (e.g. Yes = 1, No = 0). If forms are precoded in this manner it is not necessary to transfer the value to the right-hand column, as this may introduce transcription errors.

In qualitative research, in which data are presented as transcriptions of interviews or group sessions, coding may take a different approach. One of the strengths of this type of research is that by coding the data after collection the influence of researcher bias is limited. An in-depth discussion of open coding procedures is beyond the scope of this book and is covered in the literature on grounded theory and other qualitative methods (Dey 1993, Strauss & Corbin 1990).

When designating codes it is also important to consider how missing values will be coded. Again, this may depend on how the statistical or analysis software handles missing values: some packages require that a specific value be assigned to represent missing values. It may also be useful to distinguish between missing responses, refusal to answer, undecided about answer, or question not applicable.

Before the data collection form is designed a list should be drawn up of all the variables that will be collected or the questions that will be asked. Although it is often tempting to gather extra data, adding questions or tests can have a detrimental effect on data quality by lengthening the collection process and increasing the chance of errors. The researcher must resist the 'shotgun' approach and be parsimonious, including only those measures or questions that are necessary to answer the research question. To decide whether to include an item, consideration must be given to how it will be used during analysis or report writing. If a purpose is not immediately apparent the item should be left out.

Focus groups may be used to assist in the development of data collection forms by helping the researcher to identify the social, emotional or behavioural constructs that will need to be included in the measurement tool.

Once the data collection form or questionnaire has been designed, a series of pretests is recommended. For data collection forms this may be accomplished during pilot studies or the dress rehearsal (see p. 89–90). For questionnaires it is valuable to seek the opinion of someone with experience in designing questionnaires, and to trial the questions with individuals from the target population (focus group) to check for ambiguity and problems with terminology or wording. Adequate pretesting of forms and questionnaires will safeguard the quality of the data collected.

MONITORING DATA QUALITY

The goal of all data collection is to obtain complete and accurate data so that the results of the study are a true reflection of the intended population.

Data collection generally involves at least two stages: obtaining the information from the subject and entering it into the computer (small projects involving simple data and some qualitative approaches may not require the use of a computer). Often there is also a third stage, in which raw data are reduced to a single value to act as the desired dependent variable. Each of these steps provides opportunities for error. Consequently the researcher needs to employ strategies to maintain quality data at each step. Figure 12.1 illustrates the procedures and decisions required to assess data quality.

Most data will be either entered on to precoded forms/questionnaires or into a precoded computer database, or be captured as an analogue or digital signal or image. The latter category includes video tapes, audio tapes, strip charts, photographs and numeric files stored on electronic media. Although the process for screening errors is similar, there will be slight variations in the steps taken depending on the type of data collected.

Preliminary screening takes place immediately after the data have been collected, preferably before the subject leaves. This activity should be included in estimates of appointment duration. Attention to this step will prevent time being wasted contacting subjects at a later stage to resolve missing details, or worse, having to deal with the problem of how to handle missing data. Similarly, there is nothing more frustrating than to discover *after* the subject has left that the tape recorder was not turned on, that the end of the tape was reached, or that the file was not saved. (To help prevent these problems, sample outputs should be generated at the beginning of each session.)

After an initial screening of the data quality the researcher may perform any necessary data reduction procedures to produce the dependent variables. These variables can then be entered, imported or copied into the computer data file of a spreadsheet or statistics program. Generally it is advisable to perform data reduction and entry procedures as soon as possible, so that data col-

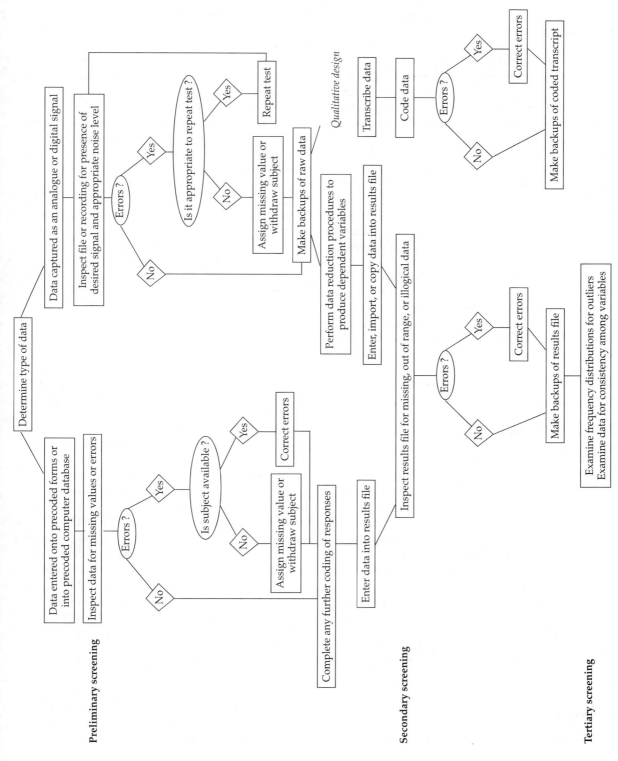

Figure 12.1   A flowchart outlining the procedures and decisions required to assess data quality

lection problems can be identified and corrected for subsequent subjects. Immediate entry also prevents backlogs and the possibility of misplacing forms. Some software programs allow the researcher to define specific validation rules for each variable, which may help to reduce data entry errors by notifying the user when the value entered is out of range, the wrong data type, or inconsistent with other values.

In the case of interviews conducted during qualitative research this step of the data management process will involve transcribing the audio- or video-taped interview to present the content in written format. This may involve a simple text editor or wordprocessor, or software designed to facilitate coding and indexing of the transcribed record.

Secondary screening involves inspecting the data file for missing, out of range or illogical data which may have been caused by errors during data reduction or entry. This may be accomplished by visually inspecting the data file or by viewing the results of descriptive statistics (such as frequency analyses) performed on each variable. Viewing the data graphically (e.g. histogram, stem and leaf plot, box and whisker plot) allows possible errors or outliers to be easily identified, and also provides the researcher with an impression of the distribution of the data.

If the data have been transcribed from an audio- or video-taped interview, secondary screening may involve reviewing the coded or transcribed report in context with the original to ensure that the transcription is correct. This may be particularly important if the original contained data from more than one individual (i.e. a group interview), or if a third party was involved in transcribing the record.

Tertiary screening involves evaluating variables for the presence of true outliers and for consistency among variables. These evaluations are based on the researcher's knowledge of the area, which allows them to discern cut-off points and expected relationships between variables.

Missing data

Missing data are a serious problem for the researcher as they can affect the validity and truthfulness of the study. There are three main techniques for dealing with missing data: interpolation, extrapolation and elision. With interpolation and extrapolation the missing value is estimated based on adjacent values in the existing data set. Extrapolation involves the estimation of data points beyond the existing values (e.g. estimating a missing fourth value based on the previous three values). Interpolation may be used to estimate a missing value based on adjacent points on either side. Elision involves deleting the value or assigning a missing value code. The decision regarding how to handle missing values is an important one, as a missing value in only one variable can often result in that subject's entire record being excluded from some statistical procedures. This can result in a reduction in the effective sample size or make group sizes unequal.

Identifying and managing outliers

When analysing the frequency distribution of a variable or regression between two variables, the majority of the values may be clustered together. Sometimes one or two values may be distinctly separate from this cluster: these points may represent outliers (Portney & Watkins 1993, Stevens 1992).

Outliers may be identified by considering the distribution of the variable(s) of interest. If the data are normally distributed, values which are more than three standard deviations away from the mean (z scores > 3) may be considered as outliers, as 99% of the values should lie within these boundaries (Stevens 1992). If the sample size is large (>100) a few valid observations may be expected to lie outside these boundaries due simply to chance. If the sample size is small, narrower boundaries should be considered (e.g. ± 2.5 SD) (Stevens 1992).

The detection of outliers for multivariate analysis is more complex, as a subject's scores may be within the boundaries on several of the variables but over all of the variables may deviate noticeably from the rest of the data set. Statistical procedures which calculate Mahalanobis Distance can be used to detect multivariate outliers (Stevens 1992).

There are several reasons for the occurrence of outliers. In the first instance the researcher should consider any circumstances peculiar to the outlying data point that may be responsible for its large deviation. Errors in measurement, equipment malfunction, errors in recording or data entry and miscalculation during data reduction are just some of the possible contributors to outliers (Portney & Watkins 1993). In some cases it may be possible to correct the error; in others this is not practical (or honest) and the value should be removed from the sample. Other reasons for outliers are related to the subject and the sampling technique used. In some circumstances the subject may have been inappropriately included and therefore present with different characteristics from the rest of the sample (Portney & Watkins 1993). Alternatively, the value may represent a true but extreme score, and had the sample been larger the probability of including other subjects with these characteristics would have increased.

When considering how to handle outliers the researcher must determine whether it is appropriate to retain the data or to withdraw the subject's data (or their particular value) from the analysis. This decision should only be made following a thorough investigation of the possible causes. If the source of error cannot be attributed to errors in data collection, reduction or transposition, then the data should be retained. Two analyses may then be performed, one including the outlier and one excluding it (Stevens 1992). The resultant effect on the calculated statistic should be discussed.

In qualitative studies outliers may represent an alternative perspective which may or may not be considered valid. Factors which help determine the validity of the response are sample size, the inclusion of multiple perspectives of the phenomenon being studied, and the use of triangulation. The discovery of alternative perspectives may be used to broaden or refine the sampling procedures to either reduce or increase representation.

PILOT STUDIES

Pilot studies, or pretesting, is an important part of any research study and plays a vital role in data quality management. Pilot studies provide information about the feasibility of the study and help to refine operational definitions and procedures (Portney & Watkins 1993). Pilot studies may also serve to assess the reliability or validity of the measures to be used. If so, the characteristics of the sample should be as close as possible to the target population and the sample size should be sufficient to produce reliability coefficients similar to those which would be obtained for the main study sample. Pilot studies may also be performed to demonstrate the feasibility of a study prior to application for research grants.

In qualitative research design focus groups or group inquiry may be used to help develop questionnaires or interview procedures. This is particularly true if the phenomenon being explored is not well defined in the literature, or when developing new theories. Focus groups provide the researcher with an opportunity to explore the participants' perspectives on the issues of interest and may reveal those that participants are reluctant to discuss or disclose. Focus groups may also identify issues which may have been overlooked or new issues important for further study; identify groups of participants who may be reluctant to disclose honest responses; help the researcher test potential questions; and refine interview skills necessary to investigate the specific phenomenon being studied.

The nature and timing of pilot studies (or focus groups) will depend on the scope of the project, the research experience of the investigators and the methods to be employed.

The number of subjects will vary depending on the main aim of the pilot study. In the initial stage of project planning a pilot study may be used to examine major issues of feasibility and measurement content. Here a small sample of convenience (2–5 subjects) is suitable. If the purpose of the pilot study is to test recruitment strategies, to verify that the procedures work, to improve the clarity of questionnaires, to determine the likely distribution of responses, or to test data reduction and analysis procedures, then a sample of 5–10 subjects who roughly represent the accessible population may be required (Hulley & Cummings 1988). If the data will be used to assess reliability or validity then larger numbers of subjects, who are representative of the target population, are needed to ensure adequate variability among subjects. If the sample is too small or the subjects are too homogeneous, statistical indicators of reliability (e.g. Intraclass Correlation Coefficient) may suggest that the procedure is reliable when in fact it may not be.

PREPARING FOR DATA COLLECTION

Most researchers recognize the use of the pilot study for determining intra- or intertester reliability but do not place sufficient value on the pilot study as a training ground for data collection. To ensure that accurate and complete data are collected some time and energy must be expended in preparation.

Training

Often the testing procedures that will be used to collect data require that those applying them be trained. Training may involve hands-on application using mock subjects, and needs to include sufficient repetitions to ensure that adequate and reliable readings are being achieved. If the measurement procedure involves interpretation and classification of subject behaviours, it is important to ensure that the examiners are familiar with the scale being applied. This may be achieved by using a written examination of definitions of terms or categories, or by having the examiners evaluate video-taped examples of the various behaviours. If the study extends over a long period of time it may be necessary to reassess proficiency at various intervals.

Dress rehearsal

Just as a theatre company performs a full dress rehearsal of a production before opening the doors to the public, a full rehearsal of all data collection procedures is a valuable exercise when conducting research. In addition to testing the procedures, a dress rehearsal will also give an idea of how long the measurements will take and how they may be organized to improve efficiency. The rehearsal should involve all investigators and research assistants who will be involved in the actual collection of measures. If possible, subjects from the target population, who would qualify for the study and who may exhibit some characteristics which might present problems for data collection, should be used. Other mock subjects (co-investigators, supervisors or individuals with specific expertise) may be chosen to give specific feedback about the methods and their implementation.

The dress rehearsal should include all the steps involved, from the initial contact with the subject to the production of statistical analyses. This will serve to identify problems related to subject recruitment, inclusion/exclusion procedures, subject management, measurement procedures, data collection forms/questionnaires, data reduction and entry procedures and analysis. Sufficient time should be permitted between the dress rehearsal and the actual study to allow problems to be resolved and changes to the protocols to be implemented.

Data management and quality control are important aspects of good research. The key to producing high-quality data is organization. Although some of the suggestions presented here may at first seem tedious, the effort invested in setting up management processes and being diligent during the data collection period will be rewarded when the time comes to analyse and interpret the data.

REFERENCES

Dey I 1993 Qualitative data analysis. Routledge, London
Hulley S B, Cummings S R 1988 Designing clinical research. Williams & Wilkins, Baltimore
Portney L G, Watkins M P 1993 Foundations of clinical research: applications to practice. Appleton & Lange, Connecticut
Stevens J 1992 Applied mulitvariate statistics for the social sciences. Lawrence Erlbaum Associates, Hillsdale, NJ
Strauss A, Corbin J 1990 Basics of qualitative research: grounded theory procedures and techniques. Sage Publications, London

4 Communicating research

SECTION CONTENTS

13 Communicating research

This chapter begins by arguing the need to communicate research findings. This is followed by a discussion of the various types of research communications and the issue of multiple or duplicate publications of the same or related work. The last section stresses the importance of good communication skills and identifies the relevant chapters in this book which are aimed at the development of these skills.

WHY COMMUNICATE?

The most compelling reason for communicating research findings is the need for transfer of information: to undertake a study and not convey the results is unethical. There are obligations to the institution that provided the research environment, to those who supervised or coordinated the study, to the subjects who willingly gave of their time and energy (often literally) to assist with the research, and to the community. When human subjects participate in research it is on the understanding that they are assisting with the creation and dissemination of knowledge, presenting researchers with the responsibility to communicate the outcome of their research (Cole 1994). Researchers may also have obligations to any agency that contributed funding or facilitated the study. Even if the findings are unexpected or negative (e.g. the data support the null hypothesis of no difference) it is still vital to communicate this, so that other researchers are better able to determine the next stage in elaborating the research problem.

In addition, government funding of university research may be linked to outcome; a major determinant of outcome is the record of publications. Thus, publication is of major importance to the continued funding of research. Individuals who complete research as part of a qualification have a responsibility to report that research by means other than just a thesis, dissertation or report, because the readership of such communications is generally very limited. Failure to publish findings will adversely affect the likelihood of receiving research funding. The funding body will consider a publication record as an indicator that a researcher has been able to successfully complete a research project and that the findings have been subjected to peer review (Cole 1994). Another important reason for publishing is to provide a means whereby other disciplines can become aware of the body of knowledge of a profession.

There is no doubt that there are personal gains for the researcher who publishes. These include a sense of pride and achievement at seeing one's name in print, and a track record of publication may enhance opportunities for employment and research funding. A publication record may be important in the successful application for scholarships and for entrance to higher degree programmes. There are also gains for the community, which benefits from the knowledge.

Within the therapies there are considerable bodies of empirical knowledge which have served the professions well during their formative years. However, there is a growing demand from various health agencies, who now seek validation of this knowledge using scientific methods. Thus it is not only academics who are required to publish to further their careers: health professionals must also publish to ensure the long-term survival of their professions.

TYPES OF RESEARCH COMMUNICATION

Many different types of research communication exist. Presentation of the research proposal provides the first means of communication about a study. The presentation not only benefits the researcher, who receives a peer review, but also provides others with knowledge about the planned study. When several individuals work together on a project the proposal serves as the working document, enabling communication between members of the research team. The remainder of this chapter is devoted to the types of communication available for reporting research findings. The researching therapist is required to assess which is the most appropriate means for communicating their research.

Journal articles

Journal articles are the most effective and permanent means of disseminating information to a large audience. Publication in a widely indexed journal enjoying the widest circulation should be the goal of every researcher. It is important to emphasize that few professional therapy journals are indexed in *Index Medicus* (Medline); consequently, it may be preferable to seek to publish in journals which are, as this is the major source of citations for many biomedical literature searches. Peer review provides some 'warranty' of quality. The disadvantage of some journals is that they are only read by members of a specific profession.

Thesis or dissertation

A thesis or dissertation is the single most important piece of written communication completed by the research student. However, the readership of a thesis or dissertation is limited primarily to the examiners and other researchers interested in the topic.

Research project report

A research project report is often written by an individual as part of a course of study. Alternatively, a report may be commissioned by an organization or individual requiring a study that addresses a specific question or issue. The brief (i.e. what should be investigated and the format of the report) will usually be set by the commissioning body, and the circulation of the report may be internal within the organization, or it may be made available publicly.

Hospital/institutional reports

Reports from hospitals or institutions often include titles of research projects (in progress or completed) and may also include a short progress report or abstract. Within a large hospital or institution such reports are usually read by individuals from many different disciplines, so this may be an effective means of telling people locally about what is being done.

Conference presentation

A conference presentation may be a very effective means of communicating research findings, allowing earlier dissemination as there is often a considerable time lag between acceptance of a journal manuscript and publication. However, not all conference presentations are subjected to peer review and, if published, the amount of detail is usually limited to that contained in a short abstract.

World Wide Web publication

Individuals and organizations are increasingly making research findings available on the World Wide Web. Although this provides rapid access to research for both professionals and the general public, there is usually no peer review of material so quality is variable.

Professional magazines or newsletters

Professional newsletters provide a rapid means of communicating research findings but generally are not subjected to peer review and are not cited in indexes. However, they do target the relevant group and, sadly, may be more widely read than research journals.

Book chapters

Chapters in books often incorporate research findings, but it is rare for a chapter to be devoted to reporting the outcome of a study. An author is generally invited to provide a book chapter and this method of communication is therefore available to only a relatively small number of researchers. Further, the readership is limited compared to that of a journal.

Media (television, radio, newspapers)

International, national and local media may provide a high-profile means of communicating with an audience which includes members of the general public. The disadvantages are the lack of peer review and, owing to limitations of time or physical space, it is usually possible to convey only a very limited amount of information.

The other methods of communication available to therapists include departmental seminars, continuing education seminars, special interest group meetings and seminars held for members of other disciplines or members of the public.

MULTIPLE AND DUPLICATE PUBLICATIONS OF THE SAME OR RELATED WORK

Not uncommonly, researchers will seek to publish two or more manuscripts from the findings of a single study by dividing the total work into very thin slices (a practice known also as 'salami publication'; Lowry & Smith 1992). Alternatively, a researcher may attempt duplicate publication on the same topic. The distinction between multiple and duplicate publication is often somewhat blurred (Henderson 1995). Multiple publications may be appropriate with a large-scale study, or a study which answers multiple questions, if it cannot be adequately described within a typical journal article because of the word limit imposed. For example, the findings of a large-scale research project which involved the development and evaluation of a new instrument could be reported in three articles. The first might describe the development of the instrument, and the second and third describe the findings of reliability and validity studies performed using the instrument in normal subjects and in different patient populations, respectively.

It is also appropriate to seek to publish the work in more than one place (i.e. duplicate publication) if the first source is not easily accessible (e.g. a report from an institution), provides few details (e.g. conference abstract) or reaches only a specific audience (e.g. therapists may need to publish their work in both medical and therapy journals). If the aim is to reach different audiences, the content of the two manuscripts should be modified to suit this purpose and each should include appropriate cross-referencing to the other manuscript. When submitting a manuscript to a journal it is important to inform the editors of all manuscripts on related work being submitted, in press or already published, and to indicate the essential differences between them.

Researchers may feel under pressure to obtain multiple publications from a single study in an attempt to impress appointment and grant committees. This practice will not only lead to problems with copyright, but also occupies valuable space in a journal. Once a manuscript has been received by the editor of a journal, the copyright for that manuscript is generally transferred to the journal, and it may not be submitted elsewhere or reproduced in any form without the permission of the journal editor. Writing the same or similar publications for the same audience is also unethical, as manuscripts submitted to journals should be original. Yielding to pressure to write several manuscripts from a small-scale study will usually result in individual papers each presenting such trivial pieces of information that they are unlikely to be published.

PREPARING RESEARCH COMMUNICATIONS

For the new or inexperienced researcher preparing a research communication is generally a time-consuming and challenging task. It is vital that researching therapists acquire a high standard of communication skills, as good research may be judged harshly if the standard of presentation is poor. The aim of the remaining chapters

in this book is to assist the development of good communication skills. Also included is a chapter highlighting the issues concerned with authorship (Chapter 16).

REFERENCES

Cole J 1994 Publishing or perishing. Australian Journal of Physiotherapy 40(2): 79–80
Lowry S, Smith J 1992 Duplicate publication. If in doubt ask the editor. British Medical Journal 304: 999–1000

 Further Reading

Henderson K 1995 Careful manuscript preparation maximises publication potential. Australian Journal of Physiotherapy 41(4): 237–240
International Committee of Medical Journal Editors 1991 Uniform requirements for manuscripts submitted to biomedical journals. British Medical Journal 302: 338–341

14 Writing in scientific style

INTRODUCTION

Every successful researcher must acquire the skill to produce written material which can be clearly and unambiguously understood by the reader. When writing a research communication, the aim should be to express and not to impress. The writing of research proposals, theses, journal manuscripts and conference papers is not easy. However, the skill of writing clearly is one which improves considerably with practice. A prerequisite for clear writing is, of course, a thorough understanding of the subject matter.

Many written research communications use a scientific style, the characteristic features of which should be clarity, conciseness, accuracy and the presentation of information in a logical manner. Correct grammar, spelling and punctuation are, of course, essential. The writing should be free of colloquial expressions and unnecessary jargon. Where possible, complex phrases should be replaced with single words. As short sentences are easier to understand than long ones, in scientific writing the recommended average length of a sentence is 22 words (Zeiger 1991). As a general rule, the harder the science the simpler the writing must be. Thus, the style of writing for a research communication is very different from that used for a literary work.

The purpose of this chapter is to provide some guidelines aimed at improving the standard of scientific writing in English. It begins with strategies to overcome the difficulties of actually getting started; this is followed by separate sections covering the building blocks of written communication, i.e. organizing material to ensure a logical flow of ideas, selecting the correct vocabulary, constructing clear sentences and writing clear paragraphs. Also included is a short section on the reporting of numerical data and results (including the results of statistical analyses). Later sections provide information on referencing and the use of footnotes and quotations. The final sections outline the processes of revising, editing and proofreading, and the critical review of written communications by others. The structure of individual sections of a research communication (e.g. Abstract, Introduction, Literature Review, Methods, Results, Discussion, Conclusions) is covered in Chapters 5, 17 and 18. This chapter is not intended to be exhaustive, but covers many of the errors frequently encountered by research supervisors, examiners of theses and reviewers of journal manuscripts. References to additional material are given at the end of the chapter.

GETTING STARTED

Getting started is often the hardest part of writing, and many writers confess to having 'writer's block' at some time. The task of writing a proposal, thesis or journal manuscript is often daunting, therefore writing tasks should be broken down into small manageable steps with feasible deadlines set for each stage of the process.

It is essential to set aside time and space in which to write. Most people are usually able to identify an optimal time for creativity and productivity, and where possible this should be assigned for planning and writing (see Chapter 11, p. 72–73). Ideally, such a time should be free from interruptions. Where possible, time should be set aside on consecutive days and used for planning or writing even if there is no inclination to do so. It may help to make a pact with oneself to write for 5 minutes, even if the result is only an outline or a few sentences, and evaluate progress at the end of this time. 'Writer's block' is often overcome by simply being actively involved in the writing process (Shilling 1985). Long gaps between periods of writing should be avoided as they interrupt the continuity of thought. To avoid

frustration, all the necessary information, for example references, data and drafts of any tables and figures, must be at hand before starting to write.

The draft outline

For a written communication to be clear to the reader, the material must be well organized and prioritized. The writer may be assisted in this by developing their thoughts into a draft written outline. The benefits of this are that the writer already knows the content of the work, has guidelines which ensure that the writing proceeds in a logical and organized way, and the outline assists with writing fluency by removing the writer's preoccupation with what to say (Committee on Scientific Writing, RMIT 1993). The first stage in the development of an outline is to document, in point form, the ideas to be covered. These should then be organized into a framework of paragraphs covering the different topics. Grouping of paragraphs on the same or related topics under subheadings is the next stage. The last stage is to organize these sections into larger sections under main headings. The process may also evolve in the opposite direction, with the starting point being major headings under which are filled in the subordinate ideas. Irrespective of the type of research communication, the organization of the material should be such that it tells a story.

The writing process

The writing process which follows the development of a draft outline is often assisted by first writing the easiest sections (usually the Methods of a proposal or the Methods and Results of a thesis, journal manuscript or conference paper). Writing quickly is a good way to keep the flow of ideas going. Abbreviations should be used and spaces left for words that do not come quickly to mind. With a first draft the goal is to get something written: it does not matter if sentences are incomplete and the grammar incorrect, so long as the main points and ideas have been captured.

It is strongly recommended that the following

resources (where appropriate) are readily available: a comprehensive language dictionary, a medical dictionary, a science and technology dictionary, a thesaurus and a style guide.

VOCABULARY

In scientific writing only legitimate words should be used, and they should be carefully chosen to convey precisely what the writer wants to say. Approximations are not acceptable (e.g. 'very few', 'almost all') as the use of such terms weakens a statement. The vocabulary used must be familiar to the reader. In more casual writing words are often carelessly interchanged (see Table 14.1) (Zeiger 1991): this is not acceptable in scientific writing.

Personal terms and non-discriminatory language

Although it is generally recommended that scientific writing should be in the third person or passive tense, there are exceptions. On occasions, the failure to use 'I' or 'we' may leave the reader confused as to whose work is being described, who is responsible for the opinions being expressed or who made the observations. In such instances the use of the first person is recommended, or alternatively 'the author(s)' can be used in place of 'I' or 'we'. Also, in some qualitative approaches the use of 'I' or 'we' is encouraged as it acknowledges that the researcher is a participant in the research process.

Every attempt must be made to avoid the use of words or terms which might imply bias on the basis of age, gender, race, ethnic group, family status, disability, religious or political conviction or sexual orientation. This guideline applies unless the use of such terms is central to the study. When reporting qualitative research, it is not uncommon to cite direct quotations. Quotations may require a disclaimer, for example if racist views are expressed. It is important not to label subjects by their disease or condition: it is more correct to say 'elderly individuals' than 'the elderly'. Another good example is use of the term 'individuals with paraplegia', as opposed to 'paraplegics'.

Key terms

Key terms are words or phrases used to name important ideas. A key term can be a technical term, which may require an operational definition when first mentioned, or an everyday word such as 'increase' or 'decrease'. In qualitative research, often phenomena emerge which require an original description. For example, in a study which found that students from a non-English speaking background had difficulty articulating their thoughts at an appropriate conversational pace, key terms such as 'word panic' were used to describe this phenomenon (Ladyshewsky 1996).

Key terms must be expressed succinctly and should be used identically throughout the work. The repetition of key terms from sentence to sentence, or from one paragraph to another, is a very effective means of showing a link (transition) between ideas. Scientific writing is not the place to be creative by varying key terms when denoting a topic, as this only serves to confuse the reader. For example, *Manual hyperinflation is a technique used with the aim of reinflating collapsed areas of the lung. Bagging is also used to clear excess bronchial secretions.* In the second sentence the key term 'manual hyperinflation' has been replaced with the synonymous term 'bagging', but it is unclear to the reader whether the change in term also suggests a change in meaning.

Capitalization, abbreviations and acronyms

Capital letters should be used sparingly. Official titles should have a capital letter, for example the names of universities, businesses, conferences, institutions and hospitals. A capital letter should not be used for 'the' except when starting a sentence or when 'the' is part of an official title. For example, the correct title is 'the Western University' and not 'The Western University'. Capitals may be used when referring to groups

Word	Correct meaning and example of use
Table 14.1 Correct meaning and use of words which are carelessly interchanged	
affect (verb)	denotes action or influence *The mechanism whereby snoring affects systemic blood pressure is thought to be the resetting of the baroreceptors.*
effect (noun)	a resultant condition *The effect of the patient's illness perceptions on rehabilitation was investigated.*
among	expresses a relationship of one item to a group of surrounding items *There was only one valid statistical test among those used in the analyses.*
between	expresses an intermediate position in relation to two or more other items *There were no differences in the range of movement of the wrist joint between the three study groups.*
can	denotes the ability or power to do something *The Barthel index can be used to assess disability.*
may	refers to permission or to possibility *The physiotherapy management of low back pain may include spinal mobilizations or traction.*
include	often implies an incomplete listing and is generally too vague a term for scientific writing *The behavioural inattention test includes six conventional and nine behavioural subtests.*
consist	to be made up of, i.e. a complete list *The behavioural inattention test consists of six conventional and nine behavioural subtests.*
increase	to make greater in some respect *Blood pressure increased with all three forms of exercise.*
augment	generally implies to increase by addition *The combination of upper and lower limb exercises augmented the blood pressure response compared to the response seen with lower limb exercise alone.*
enhance	to add to something which is already worthy or valuable *The beneficial effect of mobilizations on low back pain was enhanced by the inclusion of exercises in the treatment regimen.*
improve	to advance to a better state or quality, to make better *There was an improvement in quality of life in the group of subjects who received therapy.*
parameter	a measured characteristic of a population. Thus it is constant in the case considered but varies in different cases *The ages, weights and heights of the population were the only parameters of interest.*
variable	a quantity that can change in a given system *The dependent variables measured in each subject group were the length of stay in hospital and the number of days before return to full-time work.*
regime	refers to a governmental or social system. The word is rarely used in scientific writing *In this country there is a harsh regime.*
regimen	a systematic plan *Three exercise regimens were compared.*

in a study (e.g. Group 1, Group 2) or successive trials (e.g. Trial 1, Trial 2).

The use of abbreviations for words and units of measurement is acceptable provided only standard abbreviations are used and, on first use, the full word or term is given with the abbreviation, for example *activities of daily living (ADL)*. Thereafter, the abbreviation should be used on all occasions in the text, except at the beginning of a sentence or for a heading. Although capital letters are often used for abbreviations it is not necessary to use capitals for the full term (e.g. Activities of Daily Living is incorrect). Acronyms (e.g. RICE: rest, ice, compression, elevation) should be used only when they are instantly recognizable by most of the readership, and after being given in full on the first time of use. Once an abbreviation or acronym has been introduced, no further elaboration is required. When deciding whether to use abbreviations or acronyms, the author should consider whether their use, i.e. in reducing space, is justified if additional time is needed to understand the meaning of the sentence. It is helpful in some written research communications (e.g. a thesis) to place a list of all abbreviations and acronyms at the beginning of the document.

Numbers, numerals and units of measurement

Local regulations for written research communications, guidelines for authors of journal manuscripts and published style guides will usually give information regarding the use of numbers and numerals within the text. Such guidelines will vary considerably. For example, some guidelines may require that numbers one to nine are written in full within the text and numbers 10 and above are expressed as numerals. Exceptions to this rule might be when expressing percentages, measurements of time (e.g. 6 weeks), degrees of movement or temperature, measures which involve abbreviations (e.g. 8 cm), scores and ratings and mixed fractions (e.g. 5/8). Most guidelines require numbers to be written in full if they appear at the start of a sentence, for example *Twelve speech pathologists were recruited to the study.*

Physical measurements should be expressed in metric units using the International System of Units (SI). This recommendation applies unless local guidelines dictate otherwise (e.g. imperial measures are sometimes used in American literature). To ensure consistency in scientific writing, when reporting data from published studies the data may need to be converted into SI units.

Reporting of data, results and statistical analyses

When reporting data, the sample size (n) must be given, any missing data identified and the alpha (α) probability (P) values for statistical tests must be included. It is important to be consistent when reporting statistics and P values: for example, all statistics should generally be given to two decimal places and P values to three decimal places. It is recommended, where possible, to give exact P values or, if the statistical analysis gives a P value of 0.000, this should be reported as $P<0.001$. The test statistic and the degrees of freedom should be included, for example $t_9=1.04$, $P=0.325$; $F_{1,391}=8.92$, $P=0.003$. When citing a P value it is important to give some idea of the magnitude of the difference (e.g. a 20% increase): a P value in isolation gives no indication of the importance of the finding. In the event that the null hypothesis (H_0) is accepted, the beta (β) probability value or statistical power should be reported.

Confusion sometimes arises as to the difference between results and data. Results statements provide the message, that is, they interpret the data. Data rarely stand alone: they are facts, often numbers, which may be presented in their raw form, summarized (e.g. means) or transformed (e.g. percentages, ratios). For example, in a hypothetical study comparing vital capacity in supine and standing, the results statement and data respectively might be as follows: *Vital capacity was decreased in supine compared to standing and mean (standard deviation, SD) vital capacity in the 10 subjects was 3.97 litres (l) (0.83) in supine and 4.71 (0.93, $t_9=4.66$, $P=0.001$) in standing.* The two statements should be presented together with the results statement given first, i.e. *Vital capacity was decreased in supine compared to standing, mean (SD) values were 3.97 (0.83) litres (l) and 4.71 (0.93) l respectively in the 10 subjects ($t_9=4.66$, $P=0.001$).*

It is generally accepted when reporting results that 'significant' or 'significantly' refer to statistical significance. Thus it is unnecessary to say *the decrease in pain was statistically significant.* However, the qualifying word 'clinical' may be necessary when reporting findings which were statistically significant but not clinically significant, and vice versa. The use of the word 'significant' should be avoided when describing the strength of a relationship between variables, as it may be confused with the statistical probability of the correlation.

SENTENCE STRUCTURE

The following sections discuss sentence structure, including verb tense, active versus passive voice, the matching of noun and verb, the placing of information within brackets, misplaced or dangling modifiers, parallel structures and transitions.

A sentence should express a complete thought. This can take the form of a statement, a command, a question, a condition or an exclamation. A sentence should be easily and unambiguously understood on the first reading (Petelin & Durham 1992).

As stated earlier, sentences in scientific communications tend to be short. It is much easier for a reader to absorb a small number of items of information at one time. Thus, it is important not to include too many ideas within one sentence, either by stringing ideas together or by talking about more than one idea at a time. For example, *In three subjects, shoulder flexion increased by an average of 20° but abduction increased by a mean of only 10°, whereas in the remaining two subjects shoulder flexion and abduction increased by 5° and 20° respectively.* This sentence is confusing and should be split into two, with the first sentence ending before the word 'whereas', for example: *In three subjects, shoulder flexion increased by an average of 20° but abduction increased by a mean of only 10°. In the remaining two subjects shoulder flexion and abduction increased by 5° and 20° respectively.*

In the following example, three sentences are needed in order to achieve clarity of expression.

Correct *The aim of the study was to compare computer-assisted learning and practical laboratory sessions for the teaching of anatomy to speech pathology students. One hundred undergraduate students were randomly allocated to attend either computer-assisted sessions or practical laboratory sessions. The teaching methods were compared using three different methods of assessment.*

Incorrect *To compare computer-assisted learning and practical laboratory sessions for the teaching of anatomy to speech pathology students, 100 undergraduate students were randomly allocated to attend either computer-assisted sessions or practical labora-tory sessions, with three different methods of assessment being used for the comparison.*

Too many short sentences placed consecutively is also a problem, as this tends to be distracting for the reader. The compromise between sentences which are too long or too short is achieved by effective use of parallel structures, transition words or terms and techniques of continuity which allow ideas to flow and sentences to relate to one another. These are covered in later sections of this chapter.

Verb tense

A mixture of verb tenses is used in research communications. Incorrect verb tense is often encountered when reading the work of inexperienced writers. The future tense is used when writing about something that is planned for the future (e.g. in the Methods section of a research proposal). The present tense is used when the author is describing their current thinking about a research problem (e.g. the Introduction of a research proposal). The past tense is used when describing something which has already happened (e.g. in the Methods section of a thesis or journal manuscript). Guidelines regarding correct verb tense for specific sections of a research communication are given in Chapters 5, 17 and 18.

The active voice

A sentence is much easier to understand if the action is expressed by the main verb. This approach avoids ambiguity and assists the reader's understanding. The active voice demonstrates that the subject, or item under consideration, is doing, has done or will do the action stated by the verb. This is in contrast to the passive voice, where the subject or item under consideration is acted upon. In addition, use of the active voice leads to shorter sentences because it is possible to use series and parallel structures for listing items. For example:

Active voice *Standing balance improved.*

Passive voice *An improvement in standing balance occurred.*

Active voice *During Study 1, each subject rested for 10 minutes in the sitting position, with hips and knees flexed at 90° and arms, flexed at the elbows, resting on the upper thighs.*

Passive voice *During Study 1, each subject rested for 10 minutes, the hips and knees were flexed at 90° and the arms were flexed at the elbows. The subject was instructed to rest the arms on the upper thighs. The sitting position was used during the rest period.*

The potential problems of using the passive voice (as is the case in some research communications) is an increased likelihood of unintentionally changing the meaning and emphasis of the text and of making the text unnecessarily long.

Subject (noun) and verb

Within a sentence the noun and verb must match (i.e. singular or plural), despite intervening phrases, and must make sense when used together. Similarly, a pronoun must agree in number and gender with the noun it replaces.

Correct *The weight, height and age of the subject were recorded.*

Incorrect *The weight, height and age of the subject was recorded.*

Correct *The intervention group improved in its ability to transfer appropriately.*

Incorrect *The intervention group improved in their ability to transfer appropriately.*

Split infinitives

Split infinitives are widely used in speech (for example *It is essential to carefully follow the instructions provided)*, and although it is generally recommended that their use be avoided in written communications, on occasions this leads to a sentence that sounds very unnatural and contorted.

Information in brackets

The main use of round brackets (parentheses) is to set apart information (e.g. explanations, examples) which is not essential to the meaning of the sentence. Thus, a sentence should still make sense if the reader skips over the information in parentheses. In the following example the placing of material in parentheses changes the intended meaning of the sentence: *The response was similar in males and females (aged 21–30 years). Males in the 31–40, 41–50 and 51–60 age range had a greater response than females of the same ages.* What is clear on reading the whole sentence (i.e. including the information in parentheses) is that the response was greater in males than females. This finding occurred except when comparing males and females in the youngest age group.

Round brackets are commonly used to enclose values which represent standard deviations, abbreviations which follow the full word or term, and numbers or letters which indicate items in a list, for example *The most important parts of this communication are: 1) the methods used, 2) the findings of the study and 3) the recommendations for further research.*

Common uses of square brackets are to mark insertions in quoted text by a person other than the author of the original text and to add clarifying words without which the meaning of a sentence is ambiguous.

Misplaced or dangling modifiers

A modifier can be a word, a phrase or a clause, and is a part of a sentence that gives more detail about, describes or limits some other part of the sentence. A modifier must be accurately placed within a sentence to avoid ambiguity. The term 'dangling modifier' is used to describe a modifier which is so placed in the sentence that it encourages the reader to relate it to the wrong element in the sentence. Dangling modifiers are more likely to occur when the passive voice is used. An amusing example appears in the following sentence: *Having now been repaired, the patient was positioned on the plinth and therapy commenced.* The revised sentence makes clear that it was the plinth and not the patient that was repaired: *Following repair of the plinth, the patient was positioned on the plinth and therapy commenced.*

Parallel structures

The term 'parallel structure' means the use of a similar form for expressing ideas, either as a pair or a series, that are equal in importance and logic. This approach prepares the reader for the next idea, thereby enabling them to concentrate all their attention on the ideas and not on the form. Parallel structures are used to put together contrasting ideas, similar ideas and alternative ideas, and to make comparisons. They are used within the same sentence and for several sentences within a paragraph. A parallel structure is developed within a sentence by the consistent use, following the lead in to the sentence, of a verb, noun, adjective or pronoun (Lister 1989). The following example lacks a parallel structure:

Subjects had their weights measured using scales. A stadiometer was used to measure heights.

The information is presented more succinctly by the use of a parallel structure:

Subjects were weighed using scales and had their heights measured using a stadiometer.

Other examples of the use of parallel structures are:

Data were analysed using either parametric or non-parametric tests depending on the distribution of the data.

The aim of the therapy was to increase clients' knowledge of their condition and to improve compliance with therapy.

When writing comparisons, common errors encountered are the overuse of 'compared to'. This term should not be used when the sentence contains a comparative term such as higher, greater, less than or lower. For example:

Correct *In the age group 40–50 years, total days absent from work were higher than in the 25–39 age group.*

Incorrect *In the 40–50-year age group, total days absent from work were higher when compared to the 25–39 age group.*

Another error is the comparison of unlike ideas or items, for example:

Correct *These findings are similar to the findings of earlier studies.*

Incorrect *These findings are similar to earlier studies.*

When listing items, consistency in style is necessary. In the following example, each idea that follows the lead in to the sentence begins with a noun.

Occupational therapists were accepted into the association because of their (i) ability to provide treatment for clients with a wide range of conditions, (ii) professional approach to dealing with clients and other professionals and (iii) commitment to research and to continuing education.

Transitions

A transition is a word or phrase used to indicate logical relationships both within sentences and between sentences to guide the reader's understanding. Transitions may provide time links (e.g. since, then, next, after), cause and effect links (e.g. therefore, consequently, as a result of, hence), contrast links (e.g. however, although, whereas, consequently) or links by addition (e.g. furthermore, in addition, similarly). When transitions are used to link sentences they should be placed at the beginning of the sentence to prepare the reader for the logic of the idea that is to follow. For example, the use of 'furthermore' at the start of the sentence tells the reader that an additional idea will be presented.

Unclear transitions frequently occur when words such as 'these are' or 'it is' are used at the beginning of a sentence, for example: *Hypertension is an established risk factor for the development of ischaemic heart disease. It is also present in many patients who develop stroke.* In this examples is not clear whether 'it' refers to hypertension or ischaemic heart disease. The inclusion of the respective noun from the previous sentence is usually necessary to prevent ambiguity.

Some transitions are adverbs, for example 'also' 'this' and 'however'. Such adverbs must be placed next to the verbs they modify, for example, *The patient was also able to transfer from the bed to the chair* is clearer than *Also the patient was able to transfer from the bed to the chair.*

PARAGRAPH STRUCTURE

A paragraph is a functional unit which contains related information in a structured order. The important qualities of a paragraph that successfully communicates information to a reader are (Petelin & Durham 1992):

- Completeness – all the information needed by the reader is included
- Unification – the paragraph is organized around a central idea and has a consistent tone and point of view
- Order – there is a pattern which is logical and makes sense to the reader.

Each paragraph should tell a story. This requires organization of the ideas within the paragraph and continuity of ideas, i.e. the relationship between the ideas must be clear. A paragraph generally has a topic sentence which gives an overview of the information in the paragraph. This is followed by supporting sentences organized in a logical manner. These are used to say something specific about the topic or point stated in the topic sentence. Some paragraphs have more than one topic sentence: for example, a paragraph may begin with a topic sentence and conclude with another topic sentence stating or restating the point, or a sentence linking the paragraph to the next one. The following are examples of common patterns developed within paragraphs: cause and effect, problem and solution, question and answer, analogy, comparison and contrast, description, process, definition, example or illustration and classification. The following example uses the problem and solution approach for structuring a paragraph:

The therapist to patient ratio is unacceptably low in the rehabilitation centre. To cover the patient case load, the four therapists employed in the centre are each required to work an average of 7 hours' overtime per week. It is proposed in the near future to reallocate therapists from the acute care hospital to the rehabilitation centre. Estimates of therapists' workload in the acute care hospital suggest this decrease in staff would lead to an average of only 3 hours of overtime each week. This is seen as a temporary solution until funding for more therapists is obtained.

In this example, after stating the problem the solution is given and explained. It would be insufficient to say *The therapist to patient ratio is unacceptably low in the rehabilitation centre. It is proposed in the near future to reallocate therapists from the acute care hospital to the rehabilitation centre.* In the second example no rationale or evidence is provided in support of the statement that workload is too high or why the reallocation of therapists is a reasonable short-term solution.

Techniques of continuity

The smooth flow of ideas from one sentence to another and from paragraph to paragraph is essential. With good continuity the need for each sentence and its position within a paragraph should be clear to the reader. The prerequisites for good continuity are well organized ideas and the inclusion of all key steps in the logic (i.e. no missing ideas).

The following approaches may be used to achieve continuity: repeating key terms, maintaining a constant order, maintaining a constant point of view, placing parallel ideas in parallel form, signalling the subtopics of a paragraph or using transitions to indicate relationships between ideas (Zeiger 1991).

In the following paragraph parallel forms are used to express parallel ideas.

Following inhalation of trial medication A, peak expiratory flow rate (PEFR) and forced expiratory volume in 1 second (FEV_1) increased by 10% and 20% respectively. There was no change in forced vital capacity (FVC). After inhalation of trial medication B only PEFR increased. There were no significant changes in FEV_1 or FVC.

There are two subtopics in the above paragraph: the effects of trial medications A and B. The first sentence within each subtopic (sentences 1 and 3) describes the variables that changed and are written in parallel form. Similarly, the variables that did not change are written in parallel form (sentences 2 and 4).

REFERENCES, FOOTNOTES AND QUOTATIONS

In scientific writing statements are supported with appropriate references. The synthesis of work by others is both acceptable and appropriate. However, appropriate acknowledgement or citation is essential: the absence of these constitutes the serious offence of plagiarism.

References are cited within the text and reproduced in full in a separate list (headed 'References', 'List of References' or 'Bibliography'). Several kinds of lists are used:

- Works cited – a list of all sources which have been referred to in the text or footnotes of a text
- Selected bibliography – contains all sources cited and the most relevant of other works consulted
- Sources consulted – a broader kind of bibliography including both works cited and all works consulted, including those which are highly relevant to the subject of the text and works which are of less immediate relevance.

In research communications the bibliography generally contains only the works cited. This makes for conciseness yet provides the reader with the necessary details to locate the source of the information or concept. The list of references cited is usually headed 'References'.

There are several recognized reference systems used in scientific writing. The most commonly used are Harvard (otherwise known as the author/date system) and Vancouver (number system). This book uses the Harvard system. The required system will usually be specified in the regulations provided by an institution or in the 'Guidelines for Authors' provided by the journal. The Harvard system requires the name(s) of the author(s) and the date of publication to appear within the body of the text. References are listed at the end of the text in alphabetical order by the surname of the first author. The Harvard system is the one most commonly used in theses. With the Vancouver system, numbers are used to indicate that a reference is being used. The numbers may be given in superscript or normal style, and may be placed within parentheses, for example: *Findings of previous studies indicate that the test of visual perceptual skills (TVPS) may be useful when screening for visual perceptual impairments in adults following cerebrovascular accident.*[1,2] With the Vancouver system the references are listed at the end of the document, in numerical order, as the numbers appeared within the text. Journals

sometimes use the Vancouver system because it takes up less space and the reading of the printed page is easier when the text is not broken up with authors' names. Whichever system is used, it must be applied consistently both within the text and in the reference list.

References cited should be the most valid and the most available. Articles in peer-reviewed journals satisfy both these criteria. Texts, unpublished Honours, Master's and Doctoral theses and some conference proceedings (those for which papers are rigorously reviewed) are also valid sources but usually take longer to find and are more difficult to obtain. Abstracts do not contain enough information to allow critical evaluation of the work. Journal manuscripts which have been accepted for publication are a valid source, but those which have been submitted (but not yet accepted) are not because they are not available for reference or for scrutiny by others. The citing of personal communications and unpublished reports or observations should be avoided. Such sources do not provide strong evidence because they cannot be accessed and evaluated. The number of references should be limited to the fewest necessary by choosing the most important, the most valid and, where appropriate, the most recent.

Referencing within the text and the compilation of the list of references is made significantly easier with the use of a bibliographic software package, which can assist in ensuring that the referencing style is applied accurately and consistently both within the text and in the references. Footnotes may be used to validate a point, statement or argument, or to explain certain aspects in the main text by providing the reader with more information. However, excessive use of footnotes can be distracting to the reader and they should be limited to occasions when the material being presented is not sufficiently clear without them. Thus, an author is required to decide whether material relegated to a footnote is sufficiently important to be included within the main text, or whether it is necessary at all. Style guides or institutional regulations will provide information regarding the format to be used for footnotes and the method of referring to them (usually by superscript numerals) within the text.

When reporting the findings of quantitative studies direct quotations are seldom necessary. Conversely, qualitative studies are often presented in narrative form. The actual words of the study participants are frequently quoted to support the points made by the researcher. The following example provides quotations from a study which looked at students who were experiencing problems when undertaking clinical placements. The supervisors of these students were concerned about the impact of a fail grade on the students' self-esteem. Quotations from the supervisors were (Drake 1995, p. 155):

'You don't want to demoralize somebody. I think that's part of being in a caring profession – you care for the people you supervise, there's that reluctance, you don't say "you're hopeless, get out of the profession". '(19/5)

'You don't like to mark people up because it makes them feel better. At the same time you don't want to squash people's feelings – so you get caught in this emotional dilemma a lot.' (11/9-10)

The previous passages show the use of the participant's own words to illustrate a category which was derived from the data. The quotations have been indented and italicized so that it is clear which are participants' words, and have been referenced by interview number and page number so that they can be verified if necessary. Using participants' words in this way is one aspect of 'thick description' so often favoured by qualitative researchers.

REVISION, EDITING AND PROOFREADING

Revision, editing and proofreading of written scientific communications are essential components of the writing process.

Revising literally means 're-seeing'. Thus, during revisions the author needs to consider the document at the macro or global level. Revision requires an examination of the overall structure and content of the document. It is helpful to have a time gap between writing a document and revising it, to allow a fresh look at the approach

and enable flaws to be more easily identified. In general, several revisions are necessary before the process of editing begins.

Editing consists of sharpening or polishing the document and thus occurs at the micro level. Editing should be done in a systematic manner, and it may help to approach the task by considering the process under the following headings: organization, content, style, format and mechanics (Petelin & Durham 1992). Assuming that a draft outline was prepared, this should be referred to in order to check that the organization of the finished document is consistent with the outline and that there is a logical flow of ideas. Restructuring will be necessary if the result does not flow. The document should be read to see whether the intended meaning has been conveyed (i.e. checking the content). Editing the style requires a careful look at paragraph and sentence construction, and the language and tone used. Format refers to the physical appearance and arrangement of the document, for example margin size, typeface, page numbering and use of headings. Finally, the mechanics refers to errors in grammar, syntax, punctuation, spelling and typography. When editing, the clarity, accuracy and thoroughness of the text must be criticized and all redundant words should be removed. The process of editing can be helped considerably with the following tools, available in many wordprocessing software packages; however, such tools should not be relied upon entirely: spelling checker (this may not be context specific and so may not identify correctly spelt words that are incorrectly used, e.g. 'their' and 'there'); grammar checker (this may flag such problems as repeated words or split infinitives); and style analyser (used to check for colloquial language, imprecise use of language, the organization of sentences and paragraphs within a document and to produce counts for the average length of sentences).

The final stage is proofreading, and this should only be carried out after sufficient revision and editing has taken place. The purpose of proofreading is to ensure that the final version of the written work is free of writing errors. Proofreading requires meticulous attention to detail and thus demands full concentration. Strategies to assist with proofreading include reading through the document using a ruler to systematically move down each line of the text; reading the document several times and on each occasion concentrating on a different aspect (e.g. consistency in the use of key terms); and reading the document aloud either to oneself or to another person who has a duplicate copy. Although some proofreading can be undertaken on an electronic copy of the document (sometimes assisted by increasing character size, line spacing or margins and/or changing the font, see Typography, p. 196–197), other strategies require a hard copy. The find and replace facility in wordprocessing packages is especially useful when proofreading as this helps to achieve consistency in the use of terms and the consistent spelling of words. Given the level of concentration required for effective proofreading it is not recommended that this task is undertaken when tired, distracted, or at a time when one expects to be interrupted. Adequate proofreading is essential: manuscripts may be rejected by journals, theses not passed and grant applications not funded because of poor proofreading.

Critical review by others

Part of the process of writing is to seek a critical review from another person or persons. There is benefit from seeking comments both from those who are familiar with the material as well as from those who are experienced writers but have little or no knowledge of the subject area. It is generally much easier to correct the work of another than to be critical of one's own writing, and receiving a critical review for the first time may be devastating. However, taking criticism becomes easier with practice. One should bear in mind that the reason for seeking the comments of a reviewer is to improve the document, and thus criticism is to be expected.

The stage at which material is given to supervisors, co-authors or other reviewers will vary to some extent on their requirements. Supervisors may ask to see an early draft of the material to ensure that it follows a suitable structure and contains appropriate content. Even though this means that editing and proofreading need not be to such a high level, it is still important to eliminate spelling and typographical errors as their presence may detract from a critical review of the content. Some supervisors may request that earlier drafts of work are resubmitted together with the revised version. This often assists the supervisor, and the writer, to more easily identify the changes that have been made.

A final note of encouragement is that writing is very much a learned skill which improves with both practice and critical appraisal.

REFERENCES

American Psychological Association 1994 Publication manual of the American Psychological Association, 4th edn. American Psychological Association, Washington

Anderson J, Poole M 1994 Thesis and assignment writing, 2nd edn. John Wiley, Brisbane

Australian Government Publishing Service 1988 Style manual for authors, editors and printers, 4th edn. AGPS Press Publications, Canberra

Burnard P 1992 Writing for health professionals. Chapman & Hall, London

Cormack D F S 1994 Writing for health care professionals. Blackwell Scientific, Oxford

Kirkman J 1992 Good style. Writing for science and technology. E & F N Spon, London

Laposata M 1992 SI Unit conversion guide. NEJM Books, Boston

Morse J M, Field P A 1995 Qualitative research methods for health professionals, 2nd edn. Sage Publications, Thousand Oaks

O'Connor M 1991 Writing successfully in science. Collins, London

Peters P 1995 The Cambridge Australian English style guide. Cambridge University Press, Cambridge

Strunk W, White E B 1979 The elements of style, 3rd edn. Macmillan, New York

van Leunen M A 1992 Handbook for scholars, rev edn. Oxford University Press, Oxford

Windschuttle K, Elliott E 1994 Writing, researching, communicating: communication skills for the information age, 2nd edn. McGraw-Hill, New York

Further Reading

Committee on Scientific Writing RMIT 1993 Manual on scientific writing. TAFE Publications, Collingwood

Drake V 1995 Problem students in clinical education. The supervisors' perspective. Unpublished Master's thesis, School of Nursing, Curtin University of Technology, Perth, Western Australia

Ladyshewsky R 1996 East meets West: the influence of language and culture in clinical education. Australian Journal of Physiotherapy 42(4): 287–294

Lister M J 1989 Writing manuscripts for a scientific journal. Physiotherapy Theory and Practice 5: 147–155

Petelin R, Durham M 1992 The professional writing guide: writing well and knowing why. Longman, Melbourne

Shilling L M 1985 Twenty tips for conquering writing anxiety. Physical Therapy 65: 1113–1115

Zeiger M 1991 Essentials of writing biomedical research papers. McGraw-Hill, New York

Preparing graphs, tables and other figures

The communication of clinical information and research findings occurs in a variety of forums. Some of the more common avenues include the scientific or professional journal, verbal or poster presentations at conferences, lectures and workshops. Generally the material presented in these situations is either written or verbal, but may also be visual. A wide variety of methods are available to the researcher to present information visually. These include the more traditional graphic elements such as graphs, tables, diagrams, illustrations and photographs, as well as more complex visual presentations using video images or computer-generated graphics and animation. These various methods may be used to demonstrate or help explain complex concepts, to add emphasis or to summarize key points, or simply to gain and hold the attention of the audience. Regardless of the type or complexity of the visual aid used, for them to be effective some basic principles should be followed.

This chapter will focus primarily on graphs and tables, as these are the most common visual aids used in research communications. The terms 'graphic' and 'figure' are used generically here to refer to graphs, diagrams, illustrations and photographs. The first section deals with the characteristics of an effective graphic and provides some general guidelines for selection and construction. This is followed by more detailed information to assist with the development of clear graphs and tables.

CHARACTERISTICS OF AN EFFECTIVE FIGURE OR TABLE

A good figure or table is one which clearly and efficiently conveys the intended message to the audience. Several characteristics of an effective figure or table can be identified. First, a good figure or table must have visual impact, balanced composition, and be suitably designed for the intended medium (slide, poster or printed material). Each medium has inherent limitations on the amount and type of information which can be presented clearly: posters are limited by size and space, slide presentations are limited by time, and printed material is limited by space and publication methods. These limitations must be considered when constructing figures and tables.

Secondly, an effective figure or table aims to support, enhance and emphasize the written or spoken text by providing additional information, or by focusing attention on specific aspects of the information. Efficiency is achieved by knowing when to use a figure or table rather than words, and by choosing the most appropriate type of graphic. Stated simply, a figure or table should be used when words would not suffice, or when a verbal description would be too lengthy. On the other hand, some information is best described by a short paragraph rather than a figure or table. A general rule when considering whether to include a figure or table in a paper or presentation is to choose the method that will be the most space or time efficient.

Choosing the right type of graphic for the situation is also important. Figures and tables are generally used to facilitate the explanation of mathematical or statistical findings or to summarize data, whereas photographs and diagrams are used to provide visual explanations to theoretical concepts, schemas, research designs or specific methods. In qualitative research tables may also be used to present participant responses using words and quotes, whereas concepts and relationships may be presented using a diagram. Often the same information can be presented using either a table or a graph. In general the visual symbolism of a graph will portray the message more quickly and may therefore be the better choice, particularly if time is a consideration. In most situations duplication of information in graphs and tables should be avoided.

Finally, the background of the intended audience must be considered. The type and number of graphics used, the amount of information conveyed and the complexity of the graphic should be matched to the intended audience.

As a general rule graphs and tables should be independent, in that they should be able to be understood without detailed reference to the text. This is achieved by using clear and comprehensive titles, and appropriate labels, legends and footnotes. As the title is a common element in both graphs and tables it will be discussed next; labels, legends and footnotes are discussed in the sections that follow.

The title (caption) is a phrase that identifies the specific topic of the figure or table. As it is a phrase it does not contain a verb (the title is given in the present tense and the verb is implied) and does not require any terminal punctuation. The title should be brief, but provide enough information to allow the figure or table to stand alone. For the figure or table to be independent of the text, abbreviations should not be used either in the title or within the figure or table unless defined in a footnote.

The title is generally placed below figures but above tables. In each case the title is preceded by a label, which is used to cite the appropriate graphic element within the text. This label consists of an identifier, usually 'Figure' for graphs and other illustrations and 'Table' for tables, and a number which is incremented sequentially: 'Figure 1, Figure 2' etc. In large documents such as a thesis the label may designate both the chapter and the sequence of the table or figure within that chapter, for example 'Table 3.1, Table 3.2' etc.

The main body of the title typically consists of three elements: the variables (X independent, Y dependent), the point or topic (T) and the sample descriptor (Z). The details included depend on the type of figure or table. For a graph or table that presents the results of an experimental procedure the general format is: T of X on Y in Z (see Examples 15.1 and 15.2).

Table 4   Summary of the ANOVA results of the effects of

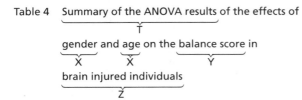

Example 15.1

Figure 5.1   The change in average torque

between days for the

trained and untrained groups

Example 15.2

Graphs or tables presenting summary information use the same elements but the format is not as restrictive, requiring only the topic (T), the names of the variables presented (X, Y) and the sample descriptor (Z) (see Examples 15.3 and 15.4).

Table N   Frequency of

use of prescription medications in

patients with low back pain

Example 15.3

Table N.N   Characteristics of medical referrals to

occupational therapy in 1996–97

Example 15.4

For illustrations, photographs or diagrams the title may contain only the topic (see Example 15.5).

Figure N   Use of an outrigger to maintain a
functional hand position

Example 15.5

The type of graph may also be included as part of the topic (see Example 15.6).

Figure N   Histogram of the distribution of the

balance score in a sample of

healthy elderly individuals

Example 15.6

In addition to these standard parts the title may also include other information. Symbols, line or fill patterns not defined in a legend or footnote should be identified and defined. Explanations of statistical information should be included, such as whether the data presented are individual or mean values and whether error bars represent standard deviation, standard error or confidence intervals. Specific features of the graphic may also be described briefly in the title (Fig. 15.1).

Titles for composite graphs should provide a general title indicating the common topic illustrated, and each individual part should be identified either as part of the main title or as subtitles (Fig. 15.2).

Although each graphic should be independent from the text, the text is not independent of the graphic and together they should form a clear sequence of information that tells the story of the paper or presentation. Consequently, the topic or point illustrated in each graphic should agree with the points stated in the text, and consistency of terminology should be maintained between the two.

GRAPHS

Graphs are symbolic representations of data, turning numbers or mathematical expressions into pictures that are more readily understood. Trends, comparisons and relationships can often be presented more effectively and concisely using a graph than with written text.

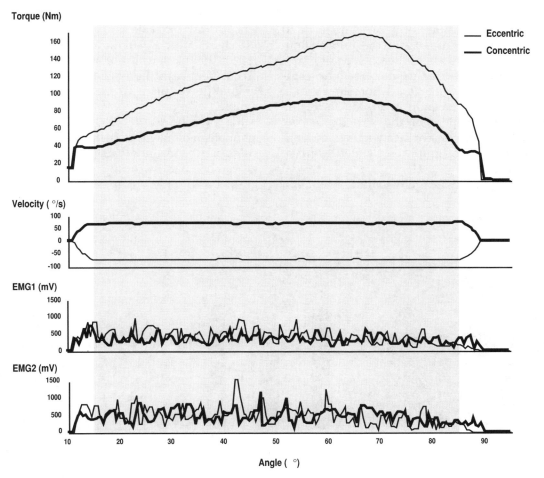

Figure N An example of the torque, velocity and electromyography (EMG) signal displays produced during isokinetic testing of the knee extensors. The grey area represents the truncated range for the calculation of average torque and integrated EMG. Torque is measured in newton metres (Nm), velocity in degrees per second (°/s), and EMG in millivolts (mV).

Figure 15.1   An example of a vertically orientated composite graph. The title includes a description of a specific feature of the graph, the use of the grey shading, and definitions of abbreviations used in the graph

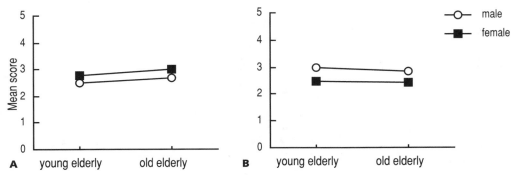

Figure 15.2   An example of a horizontally orientated composite graph in which only the left *y* axis is labelled, the *y* axes use the same scale and the legend defines the symbols used in both graphs

There are many different types of graphs, each relying on a particular form of symbolism to emphasize specific aspects of the information. The symbolism embodied in each type of graph must be understood and used correctly to communicate the idea effectively. Sometimes data may be presented in more than one form; the choice will then depend on the particular aspect of the data that the researcher wants to emphasize and the type of graph best suited to make this emphasis.

Pie charts (Fig. 15.3 A) rely on the concept of a 'whole', where the percentage of each characteristic is drawn to scale as a piece of the whole pie. Pie charts are best suited to data which seek to reflect the relationship between parts of a total. To be effective the number of divisions should be limited (fewer than 10) and the labels should be simple.

Bar or column graphs (Fig. 15.3 B) use the symbolism of height to demonstrate the relationships between values (bars projecting horizontally rather than vertically are also used). Bar graphs have only one axis on which values are

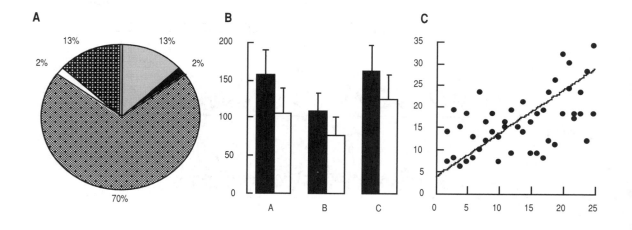

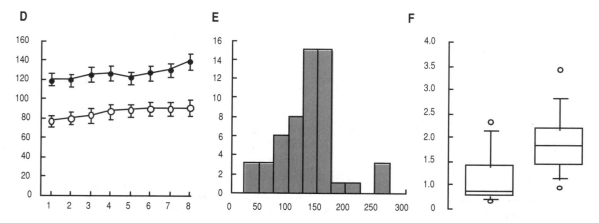

Figure 15.3   Examples of different types of graphs: (A) pie chart, (B) bar graph, (C) scattergram, (D) line graph, (E) histogram, (F) box plot. Note: titles and axis labels have been omitted

measured; the second dimension is used to distinguish between categories or groups of data.

To demonstrate the relationship between two variables a scattergram (or X–Y plot) is required (Fig. 15.3 C). As the data points in the scattergram are independent from each other they are not connected. A line or curve may be fitted to the points, however, to indicate the relationship between the variables. Line graphs (Fig. 15.3 D) depict the change in one or more variables over time, and as the values are dependent on each other they are connected by a line. The lines draw the reader's attention from one data point to the next and create an overall impression of flow, which highlights trends or relationships in the data.

Graphs can also be used to depict the distribution of a variable. Histograms (Fig. 15.3 E) and frequency polygrams display the frequency of categories or intervals of a variable, with the y axis displaying the count or percentage for each grouping. Box plots (Fig. 15.3 F) may also be used to outline the distribution of a variable by displaying the median (50th percentile), upper and lower interquartile ranges (25th and 75th percentiles), upper and lower fence values (1.5 times upper and lower interquartile ranges) and outliers.

Components of a graph

After deciding which is the most appropriate

type of graph to use, creating an effective graph involves more than just entering the data and letting the computer program determine how the graph should look. Once again the symbolism embodied in the various components of the graph is important, and choices about the composition of the graph can mean the difference between a clear effective graph and one that is not. The component that usually needs the most attention is the axes, but the symbols, lines and fills may also need to be modified to make the message clear. Figure 15.4 presents a graph as it was generated using the computer program's default values (A), and how it should appear (B). The factors which make a good graph and a poor graph are highlighted in the discussion of the various graph components.

Axes

The axis is the ruler against which the value of any point on the graph can be measured. The x axis (horizontal axis, abscissa) runs from left to right and the y axis (vertical axis, ordinate) runs from bottom to top (Fig. 15.5). Together they create a two-dimensional area on which the data are displayed (a third axis, the z axis, may be included to create a three-dimensional area on which to plot the interaction between three variables). In

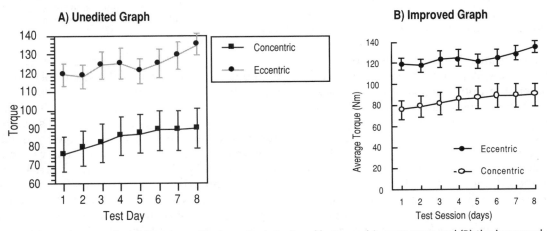

Figure 15.4 Examples of (A) an unedited graph as produced by a graphing program and (B) the improved graph after modifications were made to the axes, data symbols, legend and axis labels

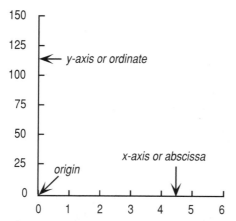

Figure 15.5 Example of a figure where the *x* and *y* axes act as rulers which mark a two-dimensional area on which data are plotted

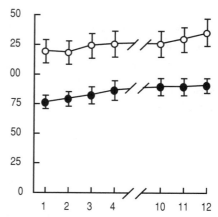

Figure 15.6 Example where break lines indicate an interruption in the sequence of data. These should be placed on the axis line and between the points in each data series to indicate that part of the series is not shown

forming this coordinate plane the axes generally intersect at zero (the origin) and have intervals of similar size.

Many computer graphics packages start the axes from the smallest value being plotted and extend them to include the largest value. Because the axes do not intersect at zero this approach can distort the visual symbolism of the graph, making small differences between points appear large. If the data of one or both variables are confined to a set of values well above zero, the axes should be broken (Fig. 15.6) or offset (Fig. 15.7), and this deviation from convention clearly indicated. Similarly, a change in axis scale (Fig. 15.8) can be accommodated using an axis break.

As most programs do not offer these options a further processing step may be required in which the completed graph is copied to an object-oriented graphics program, where the individual components of the graph can be manipulated and break lines added.

As a rule the axis lines should extend far enough to include the last data point (or error bar) and should end with a labelled tick mark. Duplicate axes which box in the graph at the top and right (Fig. 15.4 A), although often provided as defaults in graphic packages, are not necessary and tend to draw the viewer's attention to

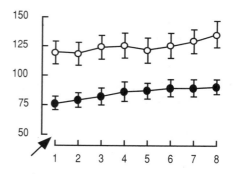

Figure 15.7 Example of where axes do not intersect at zero (the axis lines should not connect and this deviation from convention should be drawn to the reader's attention)

the outside of the graph rather than focusing it on the data. Proportional axes best display linear relationships between variables; however, disproportionate axes (*x* axis length $\neq$ *y* axis length) may be used in some instances to more accurately represent the relationship between variables while confining the graph to the desired size. When appropriate, the number of intervals displayed on each axis should be similar (Fig. 15.5). Axes should be scaled so that relationships, differences or trends in the data are presented in clinically relevant terms.

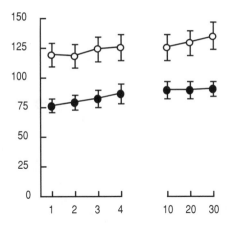

Figure 15.8 Example of two distinct axes with discrete starting and finishing points which may be used to indicate a change in scale

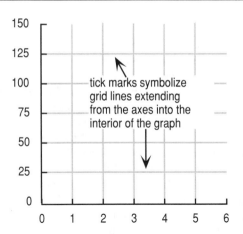

Figure 15.9 Example showing correctly placed tick marks (on the inside of the axes rather than on the outside or across the axis lines)

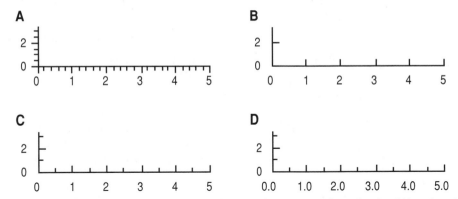

Figure 15.10 Examples of axis tick marks and value labels. Tick marks should be placed on the inside of the axes (B) rather than outside or crossing the axes (A). More increments can be designated using unlabelled minor tick marks (C). Unnecessary zeros or digits (D) should be eliminated to prevent crowding

The tick marks which mark the intervals on the axes symbolize grid lines extending from the axes (which are eliminated to prevent clutter), and thus are best shown inside the axes (Fig. 15.9). The number of major tick marks should be chosen so as to keep the axis free from clutter, using minor ticks to show more increments (Fig. 15.10 C). To allow the viewer to easily determine the value of a data point the intervals between ticks should be easily divisible using whole numbers or simple fractions (0.5, 0.25). The axis value labels should be placed outside the axis lines adjacent to the major ticks, and for numeric labels any unnecessary zeros (Fig. 15.10 D) should be eliminated to prevent crowding. If two graphs representing similar information are presented the axes of the two graphs should be scaled and labelled similarly, so that the reader can easily make comparisons between them.

Labels

Axis and line labels should give the viewer adequate information to understand the graph while remaining succinct. Labels supplement the information contained in the graph, and therefore the size, style and font should be chosen carefully to prevent distraction. The relative importance of different types of labels should be emphasized by varying the size (axis > legend or explanatory labels > numeric labels) (Fig. 15.11).

Text within labels should be presented in lower case (Fig. 15.11) with an initial capital; the use of all capitals (Fig. 15.12) should be avoided. Bold styles should also be avoided as they tend to dominate the graph and may fill in when reduced in size (e.g. for publication in a journal). Outline and shadow styles should not be used.

The font used for labels should complement the style of the main text of the paper or presen-

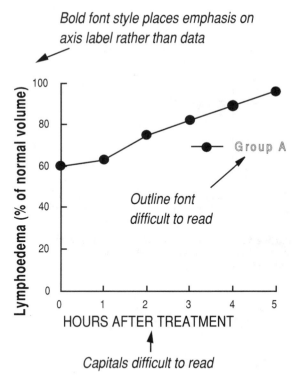

Figure 15.12 Example of a figure using inappropriate font styles

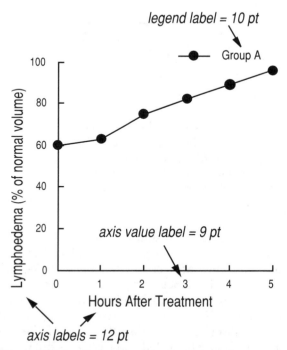

Figure 15.11 Figure demonstrating the relative importance of the various labels is denoted by differences in the font size used

tation (for journal articles a previous issue of the prospective journal should be checked to determine whether a serif or sans serif font should be used).

Labels for the *x* axis are positioned horizontally and centred below the axis line, whereas *y*-axis labels may be either horizontal or vertical and may be positioned above or beside the axis line. Horizontal labels (Fig. 15.13) are easier to read, but as they take up more space the axis proportions may need to be modified in order to fit the whole graph in the designated space. Positioning the *y* axis label above the axis or vertically beside it makes the graph more compact.

Curve or line labels may be placed adjacent to the respective line or may be grouped in a legend. Legends do not require surrounding boxes, as this tends to emphasize the legend and detracts from the main elements of the graph (Fig. 15.4 A). The legend may be placed above or

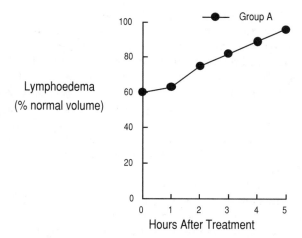

Figure 15.13   Example showing horizontal orientation of the y axis label, rather than vertically, for easier reading

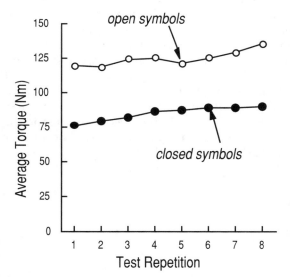

Figure 15.14   Example of open and closed symbols used to distinguish between series of data

side by side, or stacked one on top of the other. In a composite graph all of the y axes (or x axes) have the same intervals, and therefore only one axis needs to have value labels and an axis label (Figs. 15.1 and 15.2). Composite graphs are space efficient and allow comparisons to be made between graphs.

Symbols, lines and fills

Symbols, lines and fill patterns are used to distinguish one variable from another. Effective use of these requires some appreciation of the qualities of texture and contrast. Texture refers to the pattern of an object, whereas contrast relates to the differences in lightness or darkness of adjacent objects.

The symbols most commonly used to distinguish between variables are circles, squares and triangles. Contrast between symbols can be achieved by using open (unfilled) and closed (filled) symbols.

Circles and triangles are more distinguishable than circles and squares (Fig. 15.15) as squares

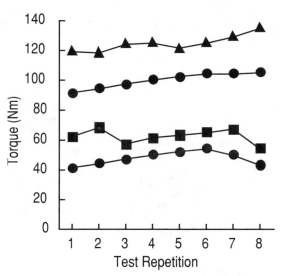

Figure 15.15   Example of how square symbols may become rounded during reproduction (circles and triangles are preferable, particularly if the data points are close together)

beside the graph, or may be included in the main area of the graph when space allows (Fig. 15.4 B). Legend symbols may also be incorporated into the figure title.

When presenting more than one graph with the same axes it may be useful to combine them into a composite graph by placing two or three

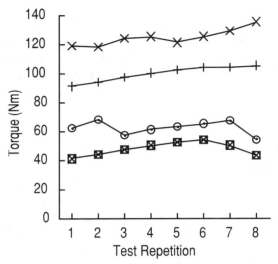

Figure 15.16   Example of how some symbols (+, X) are difficult to distinguish from the lines connecting the data points and should be avoided. Open symbols with dots should also be avoided

The size of the symbols chosen should be in proportion to the other elements and the priorities of the graph. For instance, in a line graph the lines and the symbols together present the visual symbolism of change or flow, and therefore the symbols should not be so large as to overshadow the connecting lines. Similarly, the size of the symbols used to present data in a scattergram will depend on the number of data points and the density of the spread. If the data points are clustered together, large symbols should be replaced with smaller ones so that individual points are more easily distinguishable (Fig. 15.17). The size of the symbols may also need to be adjusted to maintain balance between the different variables, as closed symbols appear to be larger than open ones, squares appear larger than circles and circles appear larger than triangles (see Fig. 15.15, in which all symbols are 12 pt).

tend to lose their sharp edges during reduction and printing. Crosses, Xs and symbols with dots should be avoided if possible. Crosses and Xs are less emphatic and may blend with connecting lines, whereas symbols with dots tend to fill in when reduced and may be difficult to distinguish from open symbols on the same graph (Fig. 15.16).

Two different techniques are available to provide emphasis or to distinguish between variables when lines are used: these are line thickness and line texture. Thick lines tend to emphasize, whereas thin lines are less prominent. When using textures with lines the order of emphasis will depend on the ratio of the length of the line and the length of the break in the line. Consequently, a solid line has greater emphasis than a dashed line, and a dashed line greater emphasis than a dotted line (Fig. 15.18). The con-

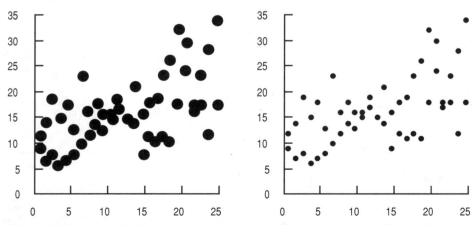

Figure 15.17   Example showing how, when data points are clustered together, smaller symbols may help to prevent overlap and make it easier to distinguish the individual points

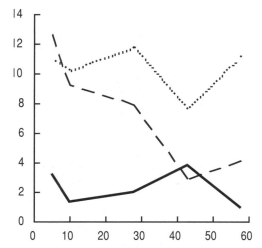

Figure 15.18   Example showing how a solid line has greater emphasis than a dashed line, and a dashed line greater emphasis than a dotted line

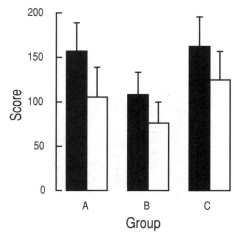

Figure 15.19   Example showing how maximum contrast occurs between black and white solid fills; black bar also tends to stand out more

trast is greatest between a solid line and a dashed or dotted line, and the difference between a dashed and a dotted line is less clear.

When presenting multiple curves, if the lines do not overlap it may not be necessary to use different line styles provided the labels can be positioned next to each line.

Bar graphs and pie charts use fills to distinguish between categories or variables. Comparison and emphasis can be made by altering the texture or the contrast of the fills. Contrast is achieved by altering the density of the dots to create different tones of grey. When using fills the greatest contrast is between black (100% density) and white (0%), and the black fill will have greater visual impact (Fig. 15.19). Adjacent fills should vary by at least 20%, but contrasts of 30% or greater provide the best results (Fig. 15.20).

The most commonly used textures for fills are horizontal, vertical or diagonal lines and crosshatching (Fig. 15.21). The line width for these textures can also be changed to create a fine or coarse texture; however, coarse textures can fill in during reduction.

Colour can also be used to distinguish between different data series. Depending on the type of graph being presented, different-coloured sym-

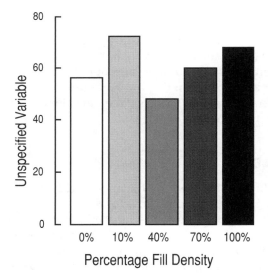

Figure 15.20   Example showing how for clear contrast shades of grey should vary by at least 20%, with differences of 30% providing the best result

bols, lines and fills may be used. Contrasting colours (such as red and green, or blue and yellow) can be used to distinguish between different data series or elements in a graph. Similarity can also be denoted by using the same or similar

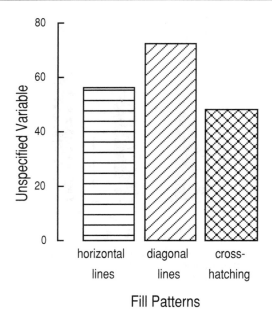

Figure 15.21 Example of common fill patterns

Table 15.1 The main components of a table

Headings		Main column heading	
	Row heading	Subheading	Subheading
Body	Subheading		
		a single cell within the body of the table[†]	

Footnotes [†] dotted borders have been used to define the borders of the cell; these lines should not appear in a table

colours (such as orange and yellow, blue and violet) for elements. Care should be taken when using colours so that appropriate contrast is achieved between the different graphic elements (bars or symbols) and between the elements and the background.

TABLES

Tables utilize the symbolism of a grid system. In a table the horizontal rows and vertical columns are used to group either numeric or descriptive information for easy viewing. Using this format a table can be used to summarize findings, group together data or results to allow comparison between groups, or to provide more detailed information to allow the reader to make calculations or draw other conclusions from the data. The purpose of the table will determine the completeness or conciseness of the information presented.

An effective table requires concise organization. To facilitate quick access to the information the design should be visually effective and incorporate symmetry and balance. As with graphs

this requires the appropriate use of the symbolism and format which define a table.

Components of a table

Tables generally contain column headings, cells, which make up the body of the table, and footnotes (Table 15.1).

Column headings

Column headings are made up of three elements: the heading label, which identifies the variable or items listed in the column; subheadings, which may further subdivide the information; and units of measurement (usually placed within parentheses). Headings and subheadings should be clear and concise, but the use of abbreviations should be avoided unless absolutely necessary, in which case they must be defined in a footnote. Bold type styles or capitals may be used to distinguish the main headings from the subheadings, but the format should be consistent across the table for headings of the same level (Table 15.1).

When presenting data or summary information the independent variables usually occupy the leftmost columns (Facility type and Gender in Table 15.2) and the dependent variables the remaining columns. This approach serves to group the data for ease of comparison. Although the independent variable may consist of different categories a column heading should still be provided. Dependent variables that are related may

Table 15.2 Changes in mean range of knee motion at regular intervals following total knee replacement in male and female patients treated at three different physiotherapy clinics. Values in parentheses represent standard deviations

Facility type	Gender	Range of knee motion (degrees of knee flexion)					
		3 weeks		6 weeks		12 weeks	
Public hospital	Male	67.2	(24.1)	68.8	(19.3)	98.0	(8.4)
	Female	88.0	(5.7)	89.0	(5.5)	90.4	(7.9)
Private hospital	Male	40.4	(11.0)	54.4	(15.9)	81.2	(10.4)
	Female	57.8	(12.9)	62.8	(6.7)	90.4	(7.9)
Private practice	Male	61.4	(21.7)	72.8	(9.1)	102.0	(4.5)
	Female	83.8	(4.2)	92.8	(2.6)	104.6	(3.7)

be grouped under a single heading, with subheadings used to identify each separate variable (e.g. Range of motion and Number of weeks postoperative in Table 15.2).

If more than one independent variable is used to group the information these groupings may be more easily distinguished by using different amounts of space between rows. For example, in Table 15.2 extra space is placed between the rows grouping each of the clinic types, whereas standard spacing is used between levels of the variable gender.

The body of the table

The body of the table is created by dividing each column into rows, depending on the number of levels of the independent variable(s). This creates boxes or cells which contain the data or summary information. The information is usually numeric, but cells may also contain text or symbols.

If data are numeric the values in each column should be arranged so that the decimal points are aligned vertically. This ensures that the true differences in magnitude are readily apparent. In most computer programs this is most easily achieved by using the decimal tab function. If the data require precision beyond the whole unit the fewest decimal places necessary to convey such precision should be used. Similarly, the same number of digits should be displayed for all values of one variable.

When presenting statistical information it is

Table 15.3 This table presents data similar to those of Table 15.2 but with the standard deviations positioned below the mean values for easier comparisons between columns

Clinic type	Range of knee motion (degrees of knee flexion)		
	3 weeks	6 weeks	12 weeks
Public hospital	77.6	78.9	100.0
	(19.8)	(17.1)	(7.1)
Private hospital	49.1	58.6	85.8
	(14.6)	(12.3)	(10.0)
Private practice	72.6	82.8	103.3
	(18.9)	(12.3)	(4.1)

recommended that the ± symbol be used with caution when designating standard deviation, as it may also be used to represent other measures of variability, such as standard error or confidence intervals. Alternatively the measure of variability may be placed in parentheses. The bracketed values may be placed either beside or below the mean value (compare Tables 15.2 and 15.3). The choice will depend on whether comparisons are likely to be made between adjacent columns or between rows. Placing the standard deviation below the mean value also helps to prevent the table from becoming too wide. Regardless of the method used, reference should be made in either the title or a footnote to the specific measure of variance displayed.

For readability the size of the text in a table should be the same as the main text and there should be adequate space between columns.

Extra space should not be placed between columns simply to make the table the same width as the text margins, as this will make comparisons between adjacent columns more difficult.

Footnotes

Footnotes are used to provide additional detail which, if included in the body of the table, would reduce its efficiency. A symbol is placed in the table adjacent to the element that requires further explanation; this symbol is then repeated below the table followed by the more detailed explanation (Table 15.4).

The designation of a statistically significant result is a common example of the use of footnotes. Statistical significance is often identified within the table by an asterisk (*), with different critical levels of alpha (α) probability designated as follows: * $P<0.05$, **$P<0.01$, ***$P<0.001$.

The most common order of symbols used to distinguish multiple footnotes is †, ‡, §, | |, ¶, #, ††, ‡‡ etc., or superscript Arabic letters, e.g. [a], [b], [c]. Footnotes are ordered in sequence as they appear in the table, from left to right and then from top to bottom.

Table 15.4 Initial and discharge functional scale scores for patients admitted to the stroke unit in 1997. Each task was measured on an ordinal scale from 1 to 5: the values reported are the mode and range in parentheses

Task		Initial score	Discharge score
Mobility	-PT	2 (1–4)	3 (1–5)*
Washing	-RN	3 (1–5)	4 (2–5)
Dressing	-OT	2 (1–4)	4 (2–5)**
Toileting	-RN	3 (2–5)	5 (3–5)
Grooming	-OT[a]	3 (2–5)	5 (3–5)*
Feeding	-OT	3 (2–5)	5 (4–5)

Abbreviations: PT=physiotherapist, RN= registered nurse, OT= occupational therapist
[a] some grooming tasks were scored by nurses
* statistically significant improvement in score $P<0.05$
** statistically significant improvement in score $P<0.01$

Formatting the table

Although wordprocessing and statistical software packages generally create tables with gridlines surrounding each cell, the following format is the standard format for presenting tables in scientific publications. To separate the components of the table from each other three single horizontal lines are used. These are positioned above and below the column headings and below the body of the table (Table 15.1). Vertical lines between columns are omitted.

If a large number of variables are presented in a table, such that the table becomes wider than the page margins, the table may be rotated 90° and presented on a separate page. However, this should be avoided if possible, as it disrupts the normal reading pattern and makes it difficult to switch between table and text.

OTHER FIGURES

In addition to graphs other figures may be used to illustrate an idea or concept. These may take the form of a drawing, photograph, flow chart or diagram. Illustrations can be used to describe anatomical or physiological features or processes, to describe equipment set-ups and procedures, to show pathways or relationships between ideas or individuals, and to visually represent theories or schemas. Diagrams are particularly useful for illustrating qualitative data owing to the complex relationships between ideas and the verbal rather than numerical nature of some types of data (Fig. 15.22).

Figures can be created by hand using traditional media or by using computer drawing packages. In either case, depending on the complexity of the drawing, it may be necessary to consult a graphics artist. Some advantages to using computer-generated graphics include the ability to easily modify or copy the contents and to resize or reshape the figure. Illustrations created using traditional media are more difficult to copy, and may need to be converted to a digital format (by scanning) in order to do so. Computer-generated figures can be submitted to publishers along with a hard copy of the figure; this

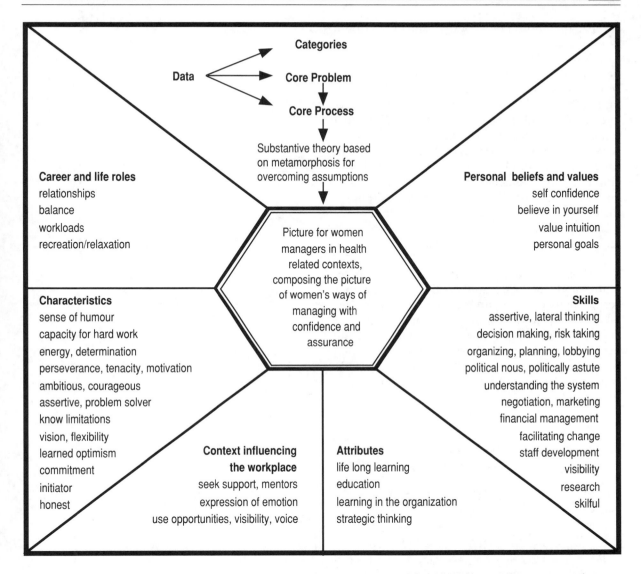

Figure 15.22   Example of one type of diagram used in qualitative research, called a 'mind map' (from Ross 1997)

allows the publisher to modify the original as required.

SUBMITTING GRAPHS AND TABLES FOR JOURNAL PUBLICATION

When submitting a manuscript containing figures and tables to a journal the graphs and tables should be submitted separately and not inserted into the body of the text. The specifications for the format of graphs and tables for a particular journal are generally presented in the guidelines for authors (see Chapter 18). These guidelines must be followed closely to demonstrate competency to the reviewers and, if the manuscript is accepted, to reduce errors during publication. Consequently, prospective authors should be careful to obtain and follow the appropriate guidelines.

The final reduction and placement of a figure or table within the text is not always predictable. Most journals make every effort to position figures and tables in close proximity to the related text, but this is not always possible. The final reduction depends on the format of the journal (one, two or three columns) and the preference of the editor and publisher. Computer technologies employed by publishers now permit graphics to be resized to suit the layout without significant distortion or loss of resolution. Graphics that are relatively square will suffer less distortion when reduced than those that are long or wide.

Visual representations of data or concepts in figures and tables can significantly improve reader comprehension. Creating effective figures and tables does, however, require some time and attention. This chapter has sought to discuss the use of various types of visual symbolism when designing figures and tables, and to provide some basic guidelines for the researching therapist to follow.

Further Reading

Briscoe M H 1990 A researcher's guide to scientific and medical illustrations. Springer-Verlag, New York

Price C 1996 How to produce clear tables and figures: Part 1. Australian Journal of Physiotherapy 42(1): 67–70

Price C 1996 How to produce clear tables and figures: Part 2. Australian Journal of Physiotherapy 42(2): 163–167

Ross M R 1997 Managerial career development for women in health contexts: metamorphosis from quandary to confidence. Unpublished Master's thesis, School of Nursing, Curtin University of Technology, Perth, Western Australia

Zeiger M 1991 Essentials of writing biomedical research papers. McGraw-Hill, New York

16 Dealing with authorship

Authorship is one of the issues that arise when consideration is given to communicating research findings. This chapter outlines some general principles for determining authorship for publications and presentations. These principles apply to all forms of collaboration, including research collaboration between students and supervisors, collaboration between professional colleagues and multidisciplinary collaboration.

There are a number of issues involved in determining authorship credit and order when a research project involves collaboration between two or more individuals. Because publications can be important for career advancement (as argued in Chapter 13), there are two potential problems which may develop: giving authorship which is not earned, and not giving collaborators appropriate credit.

Receiving credit which is not legitimately earned results in false representation of the individual's scholarly endeavours and expertise in an area, creates unfair advantage for career advancement, and potentially places the individual in a position outside their area of competence (Fine & Kurdek 1993). On the other hand, failing to give collaborators appropriate credit is unethical; it may also result in conflict and can damage both the individual's and the institution's reputation and future opportunities.

GENERAL PRINCIPLES OF AUTHORSHIP

Authorship credit is based on the notion that there has been sufficient participation in the collaborative research process by each of the proposed authors, such that each (co)author is able to take public responsibility for the contents of the publication/presentation (International Committee of Medical Journal Editors 1993). In other words, the (co)authors must have adequate knowledge of the work to be able to effectively defend it if necessary. *All* persons designated as authors should qualify for authorship ('honorary authorship' is unacceptable).

Key Point 16.1

To prevent misunderstandings and to preserve reputations and relationships it is strongly recommended that all parties involved in a research project clarify their expectations of publications and authorship. This discussion should be initiated as soon as possible in the process, and must be documented appropriately, with all parties receiving a copy of the documentation

To be able to do this, authorship should be based only on *substantial* contributions to conceptualization and design of the study, or analysis and interpretation of data; drafting the paper or revising it critically for important intellectual content; and review and approval of the final version to be published. *All three* conditions should be met by each author (International Committee of Medical Journal Editors 1993). Any part of an article critical to its main conclusions must be the responsibility of at least one author.

Authorship credit is not given in situations where participation is solely in the acquisition or designation of funding (e.g. heads of department), recruitment of subjects/participants, the collection of data, or in conducting routine observations or assessments for use in the study. In these cases, and for others whose contribution does not justify authorship, recognition should be given separately in the acknowledgement section of the paper or presentation (see p. 129).

The order of authors should be based on the extent to which each has contributed to the intellectual content of the paper/presentation.

Intellectual content refers to those aspects which define the unique contribution of the work to the scientific/clinical literature (area), including conceptualization, design, analysis, interpretation and writing (Fine & Kurdek 1993). Generally the author who has made the greatest contribution to the paper will be listed first; the remaining authors may then be in descending order based on their contributions. In some professional journals the last-named author is considered to be of greater esteem than the second author, and the order may therefore need to be arranged to reflect this. If the contribution of all authors is considered to be equal they may be listed in alphabetical order accompanied by a footnote stating that all authors contributed equally to the paper.

When research findings are presented in the public domain (e.g. at a conference or in a journal) additional information about the authors may also be provided. Details of the funding sources and the authors' affiliations (academic and clinical), in an order based upon the site of, or support of, the research project, may be included.

AUTHORSHIP ISSUES IN SUPERVISED RESEARCH ACTIVITIES

The primary example of a researcher working on a supervised research project is that of the student, but may include therapists working with a mentor or more experienced researcher. In either case the novice researcher should be strongly encouraged to submit appropriate work for publication and/or presentation at scholarly/professional meetings. In so doing, the following suggestions should be observed when determining authorship.

In general, for projects involving independent research by the student (or therapist) the student should be considered for first author position in any publication that arises directly from their research project, provided they meet the criteria for authorship stated previously. This would include honours, Master's and doctoral projects.

For projects involving a group of students (undergraduate or postgraduate research projects) the students may be listed first, followed by the supervisor, if the students have made significant contributions to the intellectual content of the project (as defined previously). Not all students in a group may meet this criteria, in which case such students should not be included as authors but should be acknowledged. The order of authorship may be determined by the significance of each individual's contribution to the paper.

In the case of projects where the supervisor has been responsible for the major conceptualization of the research question or underlying methods, has been responsible for obtaining funding (and thus has a responsibility to the funding agency to publish the findings), or is the main contributor to writing the paper, the supervisor may take first authorship. Students (or therapists) meeting the requirements of authorship should be included as co-authors, or otherwise included in the acknowledgements.

When presenting research which is the result of work towards a degree or certificate, the status and programme affiliation of each student should be stated.

ACKNOWLEDGEMENTS

Due recognition should be given to all participants in a research project. Failure to give appropriate recognition (particularly of external institutions providing support, facilities or equipment) may jeopardize the success of future projects. The acknowledgements section should include one or more statements which specify any contributions made by an individual where those contributions do not justify authorship. These contributions commonly include technical support (such as designing, modifying or constructing equipment), modifying or writing a computer program, general support provided by a research assistant or other person (recruiting participants, collecting or entering data, conducting routine observations or assessments), analysis support/advice, editorial support in reviewing or typing manuscripts, financial support or provision of equipment or materials, and general support by colleagues or the head of the department

or institution (American Psychological Association 1994, International Committee of Medical Journal Editors 1993). Each statement in the acknowledgements should specify the nature of the support given. Persons who have contributed intellectually to the paper but whose contributions do not justify authorship should be named and their contribution or specific function described (e.g. 'critical review of proposed study', 'statistical advice', 'clinical adviser', 'participation in clinical trial', 'data collection'). Permission must be obtained from all persons whose names are to be included in the acknowledgements. Some journals require a signed release from individuals who will be acknowledged.

CASE STUDIES FOR DISCUSSIONS ON AUTHORSHIP

The following case studies are presented to facilitate discussion between potential collaborators. Prior to the discussion each person should evaluate which of the collaborators presented in the case qualify for authorship or acknowledgement, the basis for this qualification and the order of authorship. Subsequent comparison between therapists may highlight different views which require further discussion.

Case 1

A group of students approached a faculty member to act as supervisor for their research project. The faculty member said they were interested in supervising the group and had a project in mind which would be appropriate. After discussion of the proposed topic all parties agreed that they could collaborate on the project. The faculty member was primarily responsible for developing the research design and methods used, the students recruited subjects and collected the data, and performed the statistical analyses as directed by the supervisor. The students wrote their research report under close supervision by the faculty member and submitted it for examination. The faculty member then decided that the results obtained were sufficiently interesting to warrant publication. The students did not feel they had the skills to condense the report and so the faculty member wrote the journal article in consultation with the students, incorporating approximately one-third of the material from the students' report.

Case 2

A faculty member and a clinician were collaborating in an area of mutual interest. A student who was seeking a project was brought into the study after the design was developed. The student was given some relevant literature related to the topic by the supervisors. The student then conducted an extensive literature search, collected and analysed some of the data, and wrote their thesis under the supervision of the faculty member. After the thesis was completed certain portions of the study were used in conjunction with other data collected and a paper for publication was written by the faculty member and the clinician. The student was not asked to contribute to the journal article.

Case 3

As part of a their responsibilities to perform research a group of therapists working in a specific area collectively reviewed the literature and designed a research project. Two of the therapists then collected the data over an extended period. These therapists subsequently moved to another service and a new therapist performed the analysis. The findings supported a change in therapeutic approach and the senior therapist in charge decided to present a paper at a national conference.

Case 4

A student enrolled in a Master's degree by thesis approached a faculty member to act as principal supervisor for a project conceptualized by the student. The student required considerable support during the writing of the proposal but conducted all of the data collection, reduction and analysis. The supervisor then recommended that the student prepare a manuscript for submission to a professional journal. The student undertook to write the manuscript but required continued support in drafting and revising the paper, which was then submitted for publication.

Decisions regarding authorship and order of authors can often be difficult. It is intended that the points raised in this chapter should form the basis for discussions between research collaborators. To reiterate: it is strongly recommended that all parties involved in a research project clarify their expectations regarding authorship as early as possible, and that these discussions be appropriately documented.

Further Reading

Curtin University of Technology 1994 Handbook of guidelines and regulations for higher degrees by research. Curtin University of Technology, Perth
Day R 1989 How to write and publish a scientific paper. Cambridge University Press, Sydney
Faculty publications and presentations policy, Department of Physical Therapy, University of Toronto

REFERENCES

American Psychological Association 1994 Publication manual of the American Psychological Association, 4th edn. American Psychological Association, Washington
Fine M A, Kurdek L A 1993 Reflections on determining authorship credit and authorship order on faculty–student collaborations. American Psychologist 48(11): 1141–1147
International Committee of Medical Journal Editors 1993 Uniform requirements for manuscripts submitted to biomedical journals. American College of Physicians, Philadelphia

17 Writing a thesis

A thesis or dissertation is a detailed discourse on a subject, and may be the sole element in a research degree or form part of a higher degree course. The terms thesis and dissertation are used differently in various countries. In some countries (e.g. Australia, the UK) it is more usual to refer to reports for Honours and taught Masters degrees as dissertations, with 'thesis' being reserved for the final report on research undertaken for a Masters degree (by research) and for a Doctoral degree. In North America these terms are reversed, with 'thesis' being used to describe an Honours or Masters report and 'dissertation' used when referring to the written report submitted for a Doctoral degree. For simplicity, the term 'thesis' has been used throughout this book.

In most cases a thesis reflects original work, founded on quantitative and/or qualitative methods, which expands and interprets available knowledge on the research question. A thesis should therefore reflect the scholarly ability of the student, their understanding of the subject matter, their ability as a researcher and their ability to think critically. The thesis should demonstrate the student's ability to define a problem, to choose appropriate methods for solving that problem, and to present and discuss the findings clearly and fairly.

The purpose of this chapter is to describe the generic issues in thesis writing. Other chapters are concerned with scientific writing style (Chapter 14) and the preparation of figures and tables (Chapter 15). Much of the content of this chapter will be relevant to the writing of research reports in general; however, it is aimed specifically at the writing of a thesis for an honours, Masters or Doctoral degree. The chapter begins by stressing the importance of complying with institutional regulations, followed by a section on the visual presentation of a thesis. The next section provides guidelines to assist with the organization of the thesis content, followed by sections providing guidelines for the preparation of the individual components of a thesis (e.g. Title page, Abstract, Declaration of originality, Acknowledgements, etc.). The concluding section to the chapter outlines the examination process.

INSTITUTIONAL REGULATIONS

Each institution will have regulations regarding the acceptable format and length of a thesis. The regulations will also detail the format of the thesis examination. The student *must* adhere to the regulations: a thesis may be returned for revision if they do not. The student should closely examine recent theses in the institution library to find examples of acceptable presentation styles.

The word limit imposed on a thesis will vary depending on the qualification being sought and the institution. In all cases the ability to write concisely is emphasized. Some examiners may refuse to mark a thesis that exceeds the word limit set. Typical word limits (exclusive of appendices, tables, figures and other illustrative matter) are: Honours thesis 8000–12 000 words; Masters by coursework thesis 15 000–20 000 words; Masters by research thesis 50 000–70 000 words; and Doctoral thesis 60 000–100 000 words.

VISUAL PRESENTATION

A high standard of visual presentation is extremely important. The term 'visual presentation' is used here to refer to the font and point size used in the text, line spacing and the style used for headings. A thesis is often a very long document and the writer should be considerate to the reader. This means choosing a visual presentation format which assists the reading and then applying it consistently.

If page margins are not specified in the institutional regulations it is important to ensure that the left-hand margin is sufficient to enable all of the text to be viewed when the thesis is bound. Browsing through theses in the institution library and assistance from the supervisor(s) will identify examples with a high standard of visual presentation. Serif fonts (e.g. Times, Palatino, Times New Roman) tend to be easier to read than sans serif fonts (e.g. Helvetica, see Typography p. 196). The main body of the text is usually written using a font size of 12 points. One-and-a-half line spacing should be used in the body of the text; single-line spacing may be used within tables, figure legends, footnotes, appendices and references. Text which has both right and left margins justified is harder to read than text in which the right-hand margin is unjustified (ragged) so, unless institutional requirements insist otherwise, right-and-left-justified text should be avoided. A new paragraph should be signalled using appropriate line spacing and not by indenting the first word.

The page numbering used within a thesis is generally Roman numerals (i, ii, iii) for all pages preceding the first chapter. Thereafter, Arabic numerals (1, 2, 3) are used throughout. Each chapter of the thesis should begin on a new page.

Chapters are usually divided into sections and subsections, with numbered headings. These divisions assist the reader and allow ease of reference. The method used to subdivide a chapter will depend on the number of such divisions and whether there are specific institutional requirements relating to this. Ensuring consistency with the style used for headings is assisted by the use of the outlining and style sheet facilities on word-processing software, which may also allow the table of contents to be generated automatically. Lists of tables and figures also can be generated automatically by some wordprocessing software. It is generally recommended that the heading levels are distinguished by font size, case (upper case, title case, sentence case), the use of bold or normal typeface and the position of the heading (centred, side heading, indented). The number of heading levels should be limited to as few as possible while still achieving clarity; for most purposes a maximum of five levels (including the chapter title) should be sufficient. An example of a system for chapter divisions and subdivisions (using five levels) is given in Figure 17.1.

It is important to provide a clear and comprehensive method of locating specific sections. The retrieval facilities commonly used include a table of contents, separate lists of tables and figures and a list of appendices. Placing the chapter name (e.g. Literature Review) in the header of each page in the relevant chapter also assists the reader to locate specific sections of the thesis. It is not usual to include an index, although undoubtedly this would be useful for retrieval purposes.

ORGANIZATION OF THESIS CONTENT

The way in which the content of a thesis is organized will depend on the research approach used and the specific studies undertaken. A thesis should tell a story (i.e. have a beginning, middle and an end), and this should be borne in mind when organizing the content. Thus it should be clear to the reader, at any point in the thesis, what stage in the story they have reached and where the next section is taking them. This can be facilitated by including, at the beginning of each chapter, a paragraph giving an overview of the content and structure of the chapter. The story line is further assisted by placing short summaries at relevant points within the chapters and at the end of each chapter. Figure 17.2 shows the layout of a conventional thesis consisting of six chapters.

A thesis describing research using qualitative methods may vary slightly from the format in Figure 17.2, the most common variation being that the results and discussion may be combined into one section, 'Findings', which may be subdivided into two or three chapters dealing with major themes. Figure 17.3 provides an example of the chapter titles for a thesis using grounded theory (Drake 1995). In this example, Chapters 4–8 inclusive present the results and discussion.

There are alternative formats which may be appropriate for presenting a thesis; one such example is a series of research publications on related topics which are collated and discussed (Fig. 17.4). This format is becoming increasingly preferred as it provides experience with manuscript preparation, ongoing peer review of the work, national and international recognition of the research findings, assists the endorsement of the research by the thesis examiners and provides the researcher with a track record in publications which may help with employment and funding opportunities. When a thesis is com-

Level 1	**1 CHAPTER HEADING, CENTRED, CAPITALS, BOLD, FONT 18PT**
Level 2	**1.1 SIDE HEADING, SMALL CAPITALS, BOLD, FONT SIZE 14 PT**
Level 3	**1.1.1 Side Heading, Title Case, Bold, Font Size 14 pt**
Level 4	**1.1.1.1 Side heading, sentence case, bold, font size 12pt**
Level 5	1.1.1.1.1 Side heading, sentence case, font size 12pt

Figure 17.1 Levels of chapter headings and subheadings

Title page	
Abstract	
Declaration of Originality / Copyright release	
Acknowledgements	
Table of Contents	
List of Tables	
List of Figures	
List of Appendices	
List of Abbreviations / Glossary of terms	
Chapter 1	Introduction
Chapter 2	Literature Review
Chapter 3	Methods
Chapter 4	Results
Chapter 5	Discussion
Chapter 6	Conclusions
References	
Appendices	

Figure 17.2 Example of the layout for a conventional thesis containing six chapters

Title page
Abstract
Declaration of Originality / Copyright release
Acknowledgements
Table of Contents
List of Tables
List of Figures
List of Appendices
List of Abbreviations / Glossary of terms
Chapter 1   Introduction
Chapter 2   Literature Review
Chapter 3   Methods
Chapter 4   Findings: Background to the problem
Chapter 5   Ambiguity: The core problem
Chapter 6   The clarifying process: Pinpointing
Chapter 7   The clarifying process: Deciding
Chapter 8   The clarifying process: Closing
Chapter 9   Conclusions: Clarifying ambiguity
References
Appendices

Figure 17.3   Example of the chapter headings for a thesis using grounded theory

Title page
Abstract
Flow chart showing sequence of studies undertaken
Declaration of Originality / Copyright release
Acknowledgements
Table of Contents
List of Tables
List of Figures
List of Appendices
List of Abbreviations / Glossary of terms
Chapter 1   Introduction
Chapter 2   Literature Review
Chapter 3   A review of the functional anatomy
                of the pelvic floor muscles
Chapter 4   Efficacy of electrical stimulation of
                the pelvic floor muscles in the
                management of stress urinary
                incontinence in females
Chapter 5   Management of urge incontinence
                using electrical stimulation in females
Chapter 6   Efficacy of home electrical
                stimulation regimens in the
                management of urinary stress and
                urge incontinence in females
Chapter 7   Discussion
Chapter 8   Conclusions
References
Appendices

Figure 17.4   Example of the layout for a thesis consisting of four papers on related topics

posed of a number of papers it is important to demonstrate to the examiners the rationale for the sequence of studies undertaken. This may be assisted by including, in the preliminary pages, a flow chart of the sequence of studies completed. When a thesis is composed of a number of papers the Literature Review (Chapter 2 in Fig. 17.4) provides a synthesis of all the topics in the thesis, including the methods used. Each paper then has its own Introduction (which serves as the Literature Review for the specific issues of that paper) and Discussion. The final Discussion (Chapter 7 in Fig. 17.4) completes the story line set up in the introductory Literature Review to the thesis.

Another alternative format may be appropriate where the study involves several more discrete elements. Each may be separated into parts and within each part the Methods, Results and Discussion presented (Fig. 17.5).

COMPONENTS OF A THESIS

The following section describes each of the main components of a thesis in the order shown in Figures 17.2–17.5. The elements which may be added to the thesis contents (not shown in Figs 17.2–17.5) include a dedication (placed after the Abstract) and a list of publications arising from the thesis (placed after the Acknowledgements or Declaration of Originality / Copyright Release).

Title page

Details regarding the content and layout of the title page should be specified in the institutional regulations. The Title page includes the title of the thesis, the name of the student, the name of the department and institution through which the research was conducted, the qualification being sought and the year of submission. Some institutions allow the student to include their previous qualifications. The Title page is not listed in the Table of Contents.

Abstract

This is essentially a brief summary (usually one

Title page
Abstract
Declaration of Originality / Copyright release
Acknowledgements
Table of Contents
List of Tables
List of Figures
List of Appendices
List of Abbreviations / Glossary of terms

Chapter 1	Introduction
Chapter 2	Review of Literature (sectioned into Parts)
Chapter 3	Part A: Exercise and fitness assessment
	Methods
	Results
	Discussion
Chapter 4	Part B: Epidemiology of osteoporosis in elderly individuals
	Methods
	Results
	Discussion
Chapter 5	Part C: Health promotion in over 65 year old males
	Methods
	Results
	Discussion
Chapter 6	Summary, Conclusions, and Recommendations for Further Research

References
Appendices

Figure 17.5 Example of the layout of a thesis separated into parts

to two pages) of the thesis. It is often the section of the thesis which is read first and may, on occasions, be the only section which is read. For these reasons it is important that the study is accurately and clearly conveyed within the Abstract. Leaving the writing of the Abstract until the main chapters have been completed should help to ensure that it is an accurate summary. A few key sentences should be selected from the main chapters to provide the outline for the Abstract.

It is important to avoid excessive use of technical terms and abbreviations and not to overburden the Abstract with detailed results; only the main findings should be included. A thesis abstract typically contains four essential paragraphs:

- The statement of the problem leading to this investigation (present tense)
- Description of methods employed – research design, subjects/participants, variables, procedures (past tense)
- Outline of the most important results (present tense)
- Discussion of key findings and implications of the findings (present tense).

Declaration of originality/copyright release

The student is required to provide a statement in which they declare that the thesis reflects their work and that all sources of information, from published material to personal communications that have been cited within the text and appendices, have been acknowledged. Recognition of any research support would usually be included in the Acknowledgements. The exact wording for the Declaration of Originality should be specified in the institutional regulations. Some institutions require the student to sign a Copyright Release statement which assigns the intellectual property of the thesis to the institution.

Acknowledgements

Acknowledgement should be made of all assistance given to the author during the planning and conduct of the research and in the writing of the thesis. This provides formal recognition of the support and shows appreciation for the efforts of others. The support may include supervision, funding, access to equipment, research space, materials or subjects, specialist advice such as technical or statistical advice, or assistance with writing or reviewing the thesis. It is also usual to acknowledge friends and family who have supported the research endeavour. The acknowledgement statement should specify the type of support provided by each individual or organization, for example: *Thanks are due to Dr John Smith of the Western University for statistical advice throughout the planning and conduct of the study.* Acknowledgement should also be given to the subjects who participated in the study.

Table of contents

The function of the Table of Contents is to provide a framework for the structure of the thesis and to facilitate the location of specific sections for reading and cross-referencing. The Table of Contents should be presented in the most informative way possible, so as to guide the reader through the work and not to confuse with too much detail. Usually three levels of headings are sufficient to provide the essential structure: more than this will crowd the Table of Contents and reduce clarity. Wordprocessing software may generate the Table of Contents with the page numbers inserted automatically. If this facility is not used, careful cross-checking is necessary to ensure that the wording of the chapter titles and subheadings is identical to that which appears in the Table of Contents and that the page numbers are correct. Figure 17.6 shows an extract from a Table of Contents in which the headings for chapter divisions have been indented; note that it includes only the first page on which an entry begins and that headings are not full sentences and so do not require terminal punctuation.

Lists of tables and figures

Complete lists of tables and figures should be included to help the reader locate such information. Tables and figures are identified by Arabic numerals, the exact title and the page number. They are also identified according to the chapter in which they are located and then listed sequentially. For example, *Table 4.3 Demographic details of the 20 subjects* identifies the third table in Chapter 4. The title of each table or figure should provide a comprehensive summary of the material presented to permit independent understanding of the content (see Chapter 15, p. 111–112).

List of appendices

The number and title of any appendices and the initial page number should also be listed in the Table of Contents. Appendices may be numbered using Arabic or Roman numerals (in upper case) or alphabetically (using upper case).

List of abbreviations/Glossary of terms

It is usual to include both standard abbreviations and specialist terms within a thesis. To avoid confusion, all key terms used in the thesis should be clearly defined. The List of Abbreviations is usually set out in alphabetical order or with subheadings (e.g. units of measurement, statis-

		page
2	**LITERATURE REVIEW**	10
2.1	Introduction	10
2.2	Importance of low back pain	10
2.3	Aetiology of low back pain	12
2.4	Approaches for assessing risk of low back pain	14
	2.4.1 Physiological	15
	2.4.2 Biomechanical	19
	2.4.3 Psychophysical	23
	2.4.4 Summary of approaches	25

Figure 17.6 Extract from a table of contents

tical terms). Acronyms must be defined completely, and preferably referenced to a standard source.

The inclusion of a List of Abbreviations or Glossary of Terms does not replace the need to write each term in full when used for the first time within the text. This includes writing the full term both in the Abstract and in the first chapter in which it is used; this is necessary because the Abstract may be read in isolation. The list should immediately precede the first chapter and serves as an easily accessible single source for the reader should they forget what an abbreviation stands for.

Introduction

The Introduction is the author's first direct communication with the reader and its content and presentation will largely determine in the reader's mind whether the thesis is worth reading. The important functions of the Introduction are to communicate the research problem and why it is significant, to state in explicit terms the research question addressed, to provide the justification for a new investigation of the problem and to tell the reader the aim of the research and the approach taken to answer the question (see Key Points 17.1). The form of the thesis Intro-

duction is more like that of a research proposal (see Chapter 5, p. 28–30) than a journal article; in a journal article the Introduction serves as the Literature Review.

The Introduction should be succinct – the recommended length is between one and three pages – and it should be written with the intention of stimulating the reader's interest. Technical terminology and excessive use of abbreviations should be avoided. It is usual to cite only a few key references which may have led to the study or highlighted the problem under investigation.

Literature Review

The purpose of the Literature Review is to provide the context for the study (i.e. to highlight why the study is absolutely necessary). The Literature Review consists of the summaries and critical analyses of reported research relating to aspects of the problem and the methods available to address it. The Literature Review should present a coherent argument, leaving the reader in no doubt about the fact that the study was necessary. This is often one of the longest chapters; however, the material discussed should be carefully selected and the temptation to tell the reader about everything read on the topic should be avoided.

By the time of writing the thesis the author may be the leading authority on the topic addressed, especially if they are a doctoral student. An awareness of this should be demonstrated in the Literature Review. This is assisted by commenting on the value of the research summarized and not merely presenting a description of previous work in the form of a list of differences and conflicts. The author's own argument should be clear throughout.

The review should be organized into sections and subsections (with numbered headings) with a short summary at the end of each major section, as this is helpful for both the writer and the reader. The review should begin with an introductory paragraph which sets the boundaries to the review and provides an overview of the structure and content of the chapter (see Chapter 5, p. 30).

Key Points 17.1

Introduction

Contents   Statement of the research problem introduced in such a way as to arouse the reader's interest (present tense)

Significance of the problem (present tense)

Research question (present tense)

Justification for a new investigation of the problem (present tense)

Aim of the research (past tense)

Approach taken to answer the question (past tense)

The chapter should be organized into the main topics or themes to be discussed. For each topic or theme, a summary and critical analysis of both the supporting and contradictory literature should be presented in a fair but critical manner. Organizing the chapter in this way helps to prevent the appearance of a mere collection of facts or opinions reported by others. Although sentences beginning *Jones reported that...* and *Davies hypothesized that...* are helpful because they make clear to the reader whose work is being discussed, care should be taken to ensure that this does not lead to a review organized article by article and not by topic or theme.

The starting point for writing the Literature Review should be a revision and updating of the review written for the proposal (see Chapter 5, p. 30–31). The review for the thesis will, however, differ from that for the proposal, as interpretation of the study's findings often requires new areas of literature to be reviewed. It is important also to update the Literature Review from the proposal stage, to ensure that all new key references on the topics discussed are included; their omission is likely to be noticed by the examiners. Additional information relating to the content and structure of the Literature Review is provided in Chapter 5 (p. 30–31) and Key Points 17.2.

The errors commonly found in a poor Literature Review are outlined in Hazard box 17.1.

Methods

This chapter describes in full the sample studied and the exact procedures undertaken to collect valid and reliable data. It is important that sufficient information is provided, either within the chapter or by cross-reference to appendices or published papers, to enable another investigator to replicate the study in order to verify the findings. This rule applies irrespective of the research approach used. The following paragraphs provide general information relating to the Methods chapter for a thesis. Further detail on the recommended content of the Methods is provided in Chapter 5, pages 31–35 and Chapter 18, pages 150–151.

The Methods should be one of the most

Key Points 17.2

Literature Review

Contents and structure	Overview of structure and content of review
	Boundaries to the review clearly identified
	Summary and critique of literature, organized into topics or themes, relating to aspects of the problem and the methods available to address the problem
	Deficiencies in knowledge highlighted
	Short summaries provided at the end of each major section
	Concluding short summary stating the current status of knowledge relating to the topic and justification for a new investigation of the topic

Hazard 17.1

Literature described and not critically appraised

Material presented article by article and not organized into topics or themes

Review reads like a collection of facts and opinions reported by others and does not represent an authoritative review

Absence of short summaries for main sections, leaving the reader unsure about the key points being made

straightforward chapters to write because it is an exact description of what the author did. Further, the outline for the chapter should be taken from the Methods written for the proposal. The Methods is written using the past tense, hence it is important to make the necessary changes when working with the outline from the proposal.

The chapter requires an introductory statement describing its content and structure, for example:

This chapter describes the study design, the hypotheses tested, the subject sample and the independent and dependent variables. A detailed description of the instruments and procedures used for data collection is provided. The main methods used for data reduction and analysis are given. Where inferential statistics were used for data analyses, the exact details of the tests are provided in the Results. The ethical considerations relating to the study are presented at the end of this chapter.

If several studies using the same instruments and procedures were undertaken, to minimize duplication it may be appropriate to assign one section for describing the elements common to these studies and to direct the reader to where the modifications are described for the individual studies, for example:

This study involved the testing of two subject populations. Sections 3.3 to 3.6 describe the methods that were common to both studies. Additional procedures used in the study of the volunteer subjects are provided in Section 3.7. Section 3.8 details the modifications to the procedures for the study of the patient sample.

It is usual to have completed some pilot studies prior to the main study and these may be described within the Methods or in an appendix; the decision as to where to report pilot studies should be made following discussion with the supervisor(s) and may depend on the purpose(s) of the pilot study(ies).

Any delimitations imposed on the study should be stated within the Methods. For example, if a sample of 20 subjects was necessary to satisfy power calculations but the limited availability of subjects resulted in only 18 being recruited, this should be reported under the subheading 'Subjects'.

Many quantitative studies will incorporate illustrations of instruments and experimental set-ups. These should be placed close to the related text and appropriately cross-referenced. At every stage in the reporting the author should describe the steps that were taken in an attempt to ensure high-quality data. For example, in an experimental set-up using a measuring instrument, the calibration data should be reported in an appendix and referred to within the Methods chapter. For qualitative studies, methods taken to

ensure scientific rigour (e.g. memos, field notes, field observations, interviews, triangulation) should be reported.

Data management and analysis

A description of the methods used for managing data (e.g. coding, data reduction) is usually given within the Methods. Sometimes it is appropriate to provide only a broad description here, with more detail being given in the Results when the data have been subjected to detailed scrutiny. The analyses used may be described in the Methods or left until the Results; they are often better placed in the Results, alongside the relevant data, especially when a large number of different methods of analysis were used.

Results

The purpose of the Results is to make sense of the data (i.e. to interpret them for the reader). In quantitative studies data are numbers which may be presented in their raw form, summarized (e.g. means) or transformed (e.g. ratios, percentages). In qualitative studies data may be words or ideas rather than numbers. There is sometimes confusion as to the difference between results and data (see Chapter 14, p. 101). In the Results, the raw data are subjected to the planned analytical procedures and presented in a meaningful way in narrative form, tables or figures. The essence is concise reporting of data and the most appropriate method for this should be selected (see Chapter 15). Data should be reported in one form only (i.e. table, figure or narrative text) except where special emphasis is required. However, narrative text should be used to interpret data reported in a table or figure. When reporting data no comparison should be made with data in published studies, as this is the function of the Discussion. Often a researcher will collect an enormous amount of data during the course of a study, and considerable time may be needed to plan the organization of the Results and the format to be used when presenting data.

The organization of the chapter content will vary depending on the study and the research approach used. The information in the following paragraphs is intended to provide some general guidelines on organizing the chapter content and for reporting the findings. Relevant information is also provided in Chapter 18, pages 151–152. Results can be reported in a thesis much more expansively than is permitted in a journal article. For example, full statistical analyses (e.g. ANOVA table) can be included in a thesis, whereas there is space in a journal article to include only the test statistic, degrees of freedom and probability (P) values.

The Results should begin with an overview of the content and structure of the chapter. At strategic places within the chapter, short summaries of the preceding information should be included to assist the reader. Results should be reported first in descriptive form, with sufficient data included to allow the reader to rework the data and draw their own conclusions. When the volume of data is too great to present within the body of the chapter, the descriptive data may be summarized and presented in a table and reference made to an appendix containing the raw data. Graphs of the raw data can be a very effective way of demonstrating major trends. The author should make a judgement about what constitutes trivial findings and not report these. However, there should be a clear distinction between what is unimportant and what fails to support a hypothesis. All results addressing a hypothesis should be given irrespective of whether they support that hypothesis or not. In the following example, the reader is told the order in which the findings will be presented.

Section 4.1 describes the baseline data for the subjects studied. The effects of the three interventions on the dependent variables are described in Sections 4.2 to 4.5. The responses are presented as raw data and as a percentage of the pre-intervention values. The results of the one factor ANOVA with repeated measures are then given.

When considering the organization of the content it may be possible to address each guiding question or hypothesis separately under individual headings. Such headings should preferably identify the hypothesis or guiding question by its content, and not merely by a number (e.g.

Hypothesis 1). If this approach is suitable, then for each question or hypothesis the descriptive data should be presented first, followed by a description of the analyses used, the findings of the analyses and the answer to the question or a decision about whether the hypothesis is rejected or accepted. Often the same data are used to answer more than one question or to address more than one hypothesis. In this case, a description of the data should be given first. This should be followed (for each question or hypothesis) by the analyses used, the findings of the analyses and the answer to the question or a decision about whether the hypothesis is rejected or accepted. The recommended method of reporting statistics, P values and the use of the terms 'statistically significant' and 'clinically significant' are covered in Chapter 14 (p. 101).

The results of qualitative studies may be presented in narrative form only, and it is common to include the actual words of the study participants to support the points being made, for example to illustrate a category which was derived from the data (see Chapter 14, p. 107). Also, with qualitative studies the Results and Discussion are often presented together and not as separate chapters.

The Results should end with a concluding paragraph stating the main findings of the study (see Key Points 17.3).

Discussion

The functions of the Discussion are to:

- Answer the questions posed in the Introduction
- Explain the findings of the study
- Compare the findings with other research on the topic
- Discuss the limitations of the findings
- Discuss the implications of the findings and recommend changes for professional practice
- Make recommendations for further research.

In contrast to the Methods and the Results, writing the Discussion requires the author to use both the rational and the creative part of the

Key Points 17.3

Results

Contents   Introductory statement of chapter content and structure

Methods of data management and analyses (either in the Results or the Methods)

Data presented in summary descriptive form

Graphical display of raw and summary data

Appropriate cross-referencing to appendices containing full data or statistical tables

Identification of primary trends in data

Presentation of significant and non-significant results according to each hypothesis or guiding question

Number of data points, test statistic, degrees of freedom and significance level included with beta (β) probability value or statistical power when the null hypothesis is accepted

Concluding summary of main findings

Information presented in a logical order (e.g. corresponding to the order used in the Methods)

Short summaries at strategic points to assist the reader

brain, and for this reason this is perhaps one of the most difficult chapters to write. The Discussion should begin with an introductory paragraph to remind the reader of the nature and scope of the study. This should be very concise and followed by a statement describing the structure of the chapter. The order of presentation of information in the Discussion should be the one which best completes the story line set up in the Introduction. Where several guiding questions or hypotheses have been addressed, the Discussion should be organized such that, following the introductory paragraph, for each guiding question or hypothesis the answer is provided followed by the explanation of the findings and

comparisons of the findings with other research, the limitations of the findings and the implications. Recommendations for further research should then be given.

Answer(s), explanations and comparisons

Answers should be given in the present tense using the same key terms and verbs used in the Introduction. Answers should be limited to the population studied.

The answer(s) are followed by explanations of the findings and comparisons of the findings in the light of existing research on the topic. This discussion should also include explanations of findings that only partially support or fail to support the hypotheses. Balanced arguments for and against the results provide the reader with an appreciation of the author's understanding of the key issues. It must be clear when the author is merely speculating or when fact or conjecture is being attributed to another author. Reasoned explanations for unexpected findings should be provided based on available knowledge and speculation. Examples of typical discussion statements which explain findings are given in the following paragraphs. The findings of the present study are reported before comparisons are made with existing research; this ordering is important so that the present study is not overshadowed by previous work.

The findings of this study are consistent with those of Davis et al (1994), who also failed to demonstrate a significant relationship between academic grades and clinical competencies in undergraduate therapy students.

This study showed that the involvement of a therapist in patient management was associated with an earlier discharge from hospital, and is in contrast to the findings of three previous studies (Jones 1991, Smith et al 1994, Yates & Brown 1992). This difference in observed findings may be due to the type of therapy provided and its earlier introduction into patient management.

The observation that males returned more rapidly than females to competitive sport was unexpected. It appeared that male patients were more motivated than females; however, there was no attempt to assess levels of motivation owing to the lack of a valid and reliable measuring instrument.

Limitations

This section of the Discussion should provide explanations for any limitations of the study which might affect the validity of the findings or the ability to generalize from the findings, and the necessary controls to avoid such limitations in further studies. The relative importance of the limitations requires comment. It is important for the author to identify limitations and not leave it to the examiner to point them out. It may be appropriate to address the limitations in the recommendations for further research.

Implications

The implications of the findings, including any generalizations which can be made and the significance or importance of the findings, should then be given. Generalizations must be restricted to the specific population studied. For example, the definition of paraplegic usually denotes an individual with a spinal cord injury affecting the lower limbs; however, the site of lesion will be quite variable and so generalizing to all individuals with paraplegia may be inappropriate when the study involved only those with a lesion below the 10th thoracic vertebra. The implications or importance of the findings can be demonstrated by describing their applications, the implications for clinical practice, or by stating speculations based on the findings. The application to professional practice can be used very effectively to demonstrate importance, for example:

The finding that earlier and more intensive therapy was associated with a more rapid return of function in the patients, as demonstrated by a reduced need for assistance with activities of daily living, and an overall reduction in financial cost, has important implications for clinical practice. These findings provide evidence to recommend changes to current clinical practice.

Recommendations

The final section of the Discussion should be

Hazard 17.2

Further analyses of data (all analyses should be covered in the Results)

Answers provided for questions which were never asked

Findings described and not discussed

Apologetic tone used when listing limitations of the study or weaknesses in study design

Endless list of recommendations for further research (e.g. trivial ones as well as important ones)

Suggestions for further research which could easily have been addressed with better planning of the study and examination and analysis of the data

Writing lacks precision, is unfocused or repetitive

Lack of a clear signal as to what is fact and what is mere speculation

Recommendations made for changes in practice when findings are not sufficiently strong to do so

devoted to recommendations for future research. These should be limited to the most important ones, and it is important to ensure that a more thorough examination of the data from the present study is unable to provide the answers.

Hazard box 17.2 contains some of the errors which should be avoided when writing the Discussion.

Conclusions

This chapter should begin by briefly restating the aim of the study, followed by the major findings and principal implications of the findings. Having read the Conclusions, the reader should be left with a sense of completeness. Information should be presented concisely: it may be in point form and the recommended length of the Conclusions is one or two pages. It is important that the link is clear between the Introduction (where the aim of the study was stated) and the Conclusions, and between the Discussion (which argues for the conclusions) and the Conclusions. The conclusions should be drawn directly from the Discussion. A common error is to present summaries of the findings and not conclusions: a summary is a brief account of what the researcher found, whereas a conclusion is a statement of the significance of what was found (i.e. what was concluded from the results). A thesis which ends with a summary and not conclusions will not have the same sense of closure to the work. The following is an example of the Conclusions to a thesis:

The main conclusions arising from the study are summarized as follows:

- *The reclined posture was selected as the preferred posture in 75% of the audiotypists studied.*
- *Speed of typing was significantly greater when the subject's preferred posture was adopted.*
- *High levels of discomfort occurred when subjects adopted postures other than their preferred posture.*
- *Although the reclined posture is recommended for most audiotypists the findings of this study showed the absence of a single 'correct' posture. This finding highlights the necessity to educate audiotypists regarding the need to adjust furniture to achieve the optimal postural support for the individual.*

References

The Harvard (author and date) system of referencing is generally used within a thesis in the health sciences. Institutional regulations may specify the style to be used (e.g. punctuation, full or abbreviated form of journal titles). Careful cross-checking of the References is essential to ensure that it includes all citations used in the thesis, including those within the Glossary of Terms or Appendices. The use of bibliographic software is strongly recommended for inserting references into the text and for compiling the References.

Appendices

A general principle is that material should be appended if its omission would weaken the presentation/argument, yet its inclusion in the body of the thesis is not absolutely necessary to the text. Material should not be placed in an appendix to overcome the problem of exceeding the specified word limit. Each appendix should be identified by a number (Arabic or Roman numerals) or a letter (in capitals) and a title. Each new appendix should begin on a separate page.

As appendices provide material which supports the main text, each appendix should be referred to at the appropriate point in the text. Appendices may be numbered sequentially throughout the thesis, or may be numbered within each chapter in the order in which they are referred to, for example Appendix 5.1 identifies the first appendix referred to in Chapter 5. If a considerable amount of data has been collected, then following discussion with the supervisor(s) a detailed summary only may be included in the Appendices, or a disk copy of the stored data may be submitted with the thesis. Examples of material which may be placed within an appendix are provided in Key Points 17.4.

REVISION, EDITING AND PROOFREADING

These important processes are dealt with in detail in Chapter 14 (p. 107–108).

THE EXAMINATION PROCESS

The submission of the thesis may represent the end of the work for the student, but the process is not complete until the examiner's reports have been received, the student has responded to the comments raised and made any necessary corrections to the thesis, the final copies of the bound thesis have been submitted and the degree has been conferred.

The thesis may be submitted either in hard or loose binding, depending on the regulations of the institution. The advantage of loose binding is the greater ease with which pages can be exchanged or added if corrections are necessary.

The format of the examination may vary depending on the qualification being sought, and will differ among institutions. In some institutions, after the examiners have read the thesis the student is required to defend it at an oral examination. In other institutions an oral defence is not

Key Points 17.4

Appendices

Contents
- Pilot studies
- Reliability data and calibration graphs
- Sample size calculations
- Advertisements or letters relating to subject recruitment
- Detailed inventory of all equipment used in the research
- Full details of lengthy calibration procedures
- Full description of lengthy procedures
- Verbatim instructions to subjects
- Questionnaires or scales
- Interview outlines
- Data collection sheets
- Coding used for questionnaire analysis
- Computer programs written for the research (unless inclusion breaches copyright regulations)
- Evidence of ethics approval
- Subject informed consent document
- Tables of raw and summary data
- Summary statistical tables (especially when numerous)
- Published abstracts
- Published papers

part of the examination process; in such instances the student will receive the written reports from the examiners and will be required to defend the thesis by replying in writing to the comments raised. The number of examiners will vary but is often two or three, and they may be internal and/or external (including overseas) to the institution conferring the degree. Examiners are selected on the grounds of having the appropriate expertise to examine the thesis, and formal approval of the examiners is usually by a committee within the responsible institution.

An oral defence of the thesis gives the student the opportunity to demonstrate to the examiners their knowledge of the research topic. It is the process whereby the student defends the way in which the research was undertaken, the validity of the findings and the significance of the conclusions and their implications. The oral defence would normally take place several months after the thesis submission, thereby allowing the examiners time to read the thesis. Prior to the oral defence, the student should meet with their supervisor(s) and/or thesis committee to discuss the structure of the oral defence and to seek assistance to prepare for it. It is also helpful to anticipate questions that might be asked and to have answers prepared. An oral defence often starts with the student giving a presentation which summarizes the thesis, and the student should arrange practice sessions with their supervisor and peers (see Chapter 19). When the thesis represents high-quality work and the student defends it well, the oral defence should be a very satisfactory conclusion to the process.

If there is to be no oral defence, examiners are usually given a couple of months to complete their assessment; however, it is not uncommon for a student to wait 6 months or more to receive the reports from all the examiners. Once all reports are in, the student and supervisor(s) are required to consider each comment raised and prepare a written response. This process must be approached with 100% attention to detail. The recommended format is to consider the comments from each examiner separately, and when responding to make clear to which section (giving chapter title, section heading, page and paragraph number) the comments relate and where any changes have been made. Some examiners will not only provide comments on the scientific content of the thesis, but may also recommend changes to improve the wording or organization of sections, as well as bringing to attention any typographical, grammatical or spelling errors, or errors in citations or in the References, which were missed during proofreading. When responding to the examiners it is important to address every comment, query or discussion point raised. Scientific integrity should not be compromised when replying to the examiner's comments and making changes to the thesis. The following paragraphs are examples of responses to the comments raised by an examiner, Examiner 1. The responses would appear on a page headed with the thesis title, the student's name and *Responses to Comments Raised by Examiner 1*. When replying to the comments, it may be necessary to cite (in full) supporting references.

Chapter 3 Methods
Calibration of pneumotachograph (Section 3.4 Procedures, page 45, para 2)
The method of calibrating the pneumotachograph has been clarified by adding the following two sentences. Calibration was performed using a 3 litre syringe to deliver a range of fast and slow flows using the method of Smith et al (1975) (see page 46, para 3). Flow signals were integrated to provide volume measurements, all of which were within 3 (SD, 0.02) litres (see Appendix 3, page 157).

Chapter 5 Discussion
Gas exchange abnormalities
The examiner suggests that the low arterial oxygen tension observed in the patients at 48 hours following surgery was due to alveolar hypoventilation secondary to the reduced tidal volume. Although it is agreed that the narcotic analgesics given to patients in the early period following surgery could have resulted in alveolar hypoventilation, the data obtained in this study do not support this. All of the 30 subjects studied had a low arterial carbon dioxide tension (see raw data in Appendix 4.6, page 280) and therefore alveolar hypoventilation was eliminated as a possible mechanism. The most likely mechanisms for the reduction in oxygen tension are the presence of ventilation perfusion mismatch and intrapulmonary shunting. The low tidal volume may have been due to the decreased lung and/or chest wall compliance and the presence or fear of pain. Section 5.4 (Gas exchange abnormalities) has been modified to make clear that alveolar hypoventilation was not present (see page 210, paras 3 and 4) and to explain further the mechanisms thought to be responsible (see page 214, paras 1 and 2).

Chapter 5 Discussion
Long-term follow-up of subjects
It is accepted that useful data might have been obtained by an additional follow-up assessment of subjects at 2 years following cessation of therapy; however, this was not feasible. The rehabilitation centre where therapy was provided is a tertiary referral centre (see Methods, Section 3.3 Research environment, page 60, para 2) to which all patients in the State requiring intensive rehabilitation following spinal cord injury are referred. Many of the subjects lived a considerable distance from the centre and it would not have been feasible to conduct a follow-up assessment. This point has been clarified within the Methods (page 61, para 4) and commented upon in the Discussion (page 123, para 2).

PUBLICATION OF THE FINDINGS

Access to an unpublished thesis is limited (i.e. tends to be restricted to interlibrary loan) and most individuals do not have sufficient time or the inclination to read an entire thesis. Thus it is of utmost importance to present the findings of work completed for a thesis at conferences, and to publish the work in an indexed journal. Indeed, failure to do so may be considered unethical (see Chapter 13, p. 93–94). It is especially helpful for a student to present the work prior to completing the thesis so that feedback can be considered and comments incorporated into the submitted thesis. Students are advised at an early stage to discuss with their supervisor(s) possible conference presentations and journal publication of their work. Chapters 16, 18 and 21 provide guidelines to assist with this process.

For researching therapists who are required to write a thesis, the experience represents a major challenge which at times may appear overwhelming. The material presented in this chapter and in Chapters 14 and 15 is aimed at assisting with the task of writing of a thesis.

 Further Reading

Anderson J, Poole M 1994 Thesis and assignment writing, 2nd edn. John Wiley, Brisbane
Drake V 1995 Problem students in clinical education.

Further Reading (*cont'd*)

The supervisor's perspective. Unpublished
Masters thesis, School of Nursing, Curtin
University of Technology, Perth
Evans D 1995 How to write a better thesis or report.
Melbourne University Press, Carlton
Mauch J E, Birch J W 1993 Guide to the successful
thesis and dissertation: a handbook for students
and faculty, 3rd edn. Marcel Dekker, New York
Rudestam K E, Newton R R 1992 Surviving your
dissertation. Sage Publications, Newbury Park
Van Wagenen R K 1991 Writing a thesis. Substance
and style. Prentice-Hall, New Jersey

18 Writing a journal article

INTRODUCTION

Publication in a widely indexed, reputable peer-reviewed journal should be the goal of every researcher, as this is the most effective and permanent means of disseminating information to a large audience. The acceptance of a manuscript will, of course, depend on the value of the research reported. However, a manuscript which lacks clarity and accuracy in the writing, or in the presentation of tables or figures, will be harder for a reviewer to understand. A poor standard of presentation is likely to have a negative effect and can easily be avoided by appropriate attention to detail during manuscript preparation. The guidelines in this chapter are intended to assist with the preparation of a manuscript for a scientific journal. The chapter begins with guidelines for choosing a journal, followed by a section discussing the structure and content of a manuscript. The importance of, and procedures for, a 'mock review' are then discussed. The final sections describe the processes of manuscript submission, the journal review process and the method of responding to comments raised in the review. Chapters 14 and 15 respectively provide important information relating to scientific writing style and the preparation of graphs, tables and other figures. Throughout this chapter the term 'manuscript' is used when referring to the document submitted to a journal; 'article' is used to indicate the published journal paper.

CHOICE OF JOURNAL

Before writing a first draft it is important to establish that the topic of the manuscript is likely to be consistent with the focus of the intended journal. This may be clearly stated within the journal or may be determined by examining a number of recent issues. Depending on the subject of the research, there may be several journals to choose from. In this case the writer may consider which is the most prestigious journal, who constitutes the readership, where the journal is cited and how long the delay is between acceptance of a manuscript and publication (see p. 155). Alternatively, there may be only one suitable journal for the manuscript.

Having selected a journal, it is essential to carefully read and follow the 'Guidelines for Authors' published in the journal or obtained directly from the editor or publisher. These are usually very specific and include rules about word limits, organization of the manuscript, title page information, margins, line spacing, preparation of figures and tables and the method used to cite references. Failure to comply with the guidelines may result in rejection or return of the manuscript for correction, thereby delaying the process of review and publication.

WRITING THE MANUSCRIPT

The process of writing for a journal differs strikingly from writing a thesis. In a journal manuscript the writer must demonstrate a conciseness and economy of words which best convey the essence of the research. The art of writing a manuscript improves with practice and considerable help may be obtained by asking others, especially those who have published, to criticize and review drafts. This also provides a second check of accuracy and internal consistency. One recommendation is to start by writing the easiest sections. These are usually the Methods and Results, followed by the Discussion, Conclusions and Introduction, leaving the Abstract until last. Strategies to assist with getting started are provided in Chapter 14 (p. 98).

Often a manuscript has more than one author

(see Chapter 16) and hence the writing can be shared. Ways in which this might occur include the first author writing the entire first draft of the manuscript and the other authors revising this or parts of it. Alternatively, different authors may write the first draft of individual sections or one author may be responsible for preparing the figures and tables. Irrespective of how the writing task is shared, the style needs to be consistent throughout, so even if sections of the early drafts are written by different authors, the first author must go through the entire manuscript and make any necessary editorial changes before submitting it.

STRUCTURE AND CONTENT OF A MANUSCRIPT

A manuscript is typically composed of a number of sections: Abstract, Introduction, Methods, Results, Discussion, Conclusions and References. In order to maintain continuity between the key sections (Introduction, Methods, Results, Discussion) it is helpful to consider the manuscript as telling a story. The strong parts to the story line are the Introduction and the Discussion, so the link between these sections must be clear. The research question stated in the Introduction should be answered at the beginning of the Discussion. In qualitative studies reporting the findings of narrative analyses, the sections may vary from the standard format. Such a manuscript may begin with some background information, followed by the Methods and then a combined Results and Discussion, often referred to as 'Findings'.

There is usually a word limit imposed on journal articles, so it is essential to be concise and economical with words. Unimportant or irrelevant information must be left out. In contrast to the style for a thesis, the sections of a manuscript must be highly condensed. For example, an extensive review of the literature is mandatory for a thesis, but in a journal article there is space to include in the Introduction only the most critical and important papers. Having invested many hours in undertaking research, the author may be tempted to tell the reader everything read and learned in the process, and to provide all the data gathered. To keep within the word limit it is essential to decide during the planning stages what information is essential and what can be left out. In the case of a large study it may be necessary to write several papers which cover different aspects of the research (see Chapter 13 for a discussion of the issues concerning multiple and duplicate publication of same or related work).

Title page

This consists of the title of the manuscript and the author details. The title provides the first impression and influences whether a reader is interested in reading the manuscript, so selecting the most appropriate title requires some thought. The title should include all essential key words in the right order so that the topic is accurately and fully conveyed (e.g. clearly related to the purpose of the study). Long titles should be avoided: the recommended length is 10–12 words. Also to be avoided are titles which begin with redundant words, such as *A study of*.

The names of each author and their academic and professional qualifications and affiliations (e.g. name of hospital, university) must be given. The 'Guidelines for Authors' will specify how much detail for each author can be given, for example some journals print only surname and first initial and highest qualification for each author. The 'Guidelines for Authors' may also ask for the current position and other biographical details of each author. Also included on this page are the contact details (e.g. postal address, telephone number, fax number and e-mail address) for the author to whom correspondence is to be addressed. Authors may also be asked to specify to whom readers should apply for offprints. Additional information which may be requested is a statement indicating whether the research was undertaken by a student (e.g. as part of an undergraduate or higher degree).

Key words

Most journals require the author to identify some key words (often between three and five, occa-sionally as many as 10) which represent the major concepts of the paper. These are used for indexing and retrieval purposes and should be selected from the *Index Medicus* Medical Subject Headings (MeSH). This is the current authoritative list for the subject analysis of medical literature. For example, 'physiotherapy' is not included in MeSH: the equivalent term is 'physical therapy'.

Abstract

The Abstract presents a brief summary of the content of the manuscript, and should provide highlights from the Introduction, Methods, Results, Discussion and Conclusions. Some journals require authors to write the Abstract in a structured format under set headings, for example: Background and Purpose, Subjects, Methods, Results, Conclusions and Discussion. There is often a specified word limit for the Abstract (e.g. 200–250 words).

The Abstract must make sense when read in isolation for those who do not read the rest of the manuscript. This is especially important given that many computerized searches also retrieve the Abstract. The Abstract must also be a clear and accurate recapitulation of the manuscript for readers who read the entire article: for example, it must not contain data which are not included in the Results. A summary of the contents of the Abstract is presented in Key Points 18.1.

The Abstract is usually written as one or two paragraphs, and it is important that the text flows and is not just a collection of disjointed sentences. The choice of words should be simple, jargon avoided and abbreviations omitted, except for standard units of measurement and statistical terms. Citations are not usually included. Excessive detail is unacceptable, for example long lists of variables, large amounts of data or an excessive number of probability (P) values. Journal style will vary as to whether statistical results are included or omitted from the Abstract. The art of producing a clear abstract is to provide just enough detail to demonstrate that the design of the study was good and that the evidence for the answer to the question is strong.

Key Points 18.1

Abstract	
Contents	
The problem	One or two sentences of background information
Methods	Clear statement of the question asked and why (present tense)
	What was done to answer the question (past tense) – research design, population studied, independent and dependent variables (when appropriate)
Results	Findings that answer the question (past tense) – the most important results and evidence (data) presented in a logical order
Conclusion	The answer to the question (present tense)
	An implication or a speculation based on the answer (present tense)

Key Points 18.2

Introduction	
Contents	
Background	Background to the topic (past tense)
	What is known or believed about the topic
	What is still unknown or problematic
	Findings of relevant studies (past tense)
	Importance of the topic
Question	Statement of the research question
	Several ways can be used to signal the research question, for example
	To determine whether …
	The purpose of this study was to …
	This study tested the hypothesis that …
	This study was undertaken to …
Approach	Approach taken to answer the question (past tense)

Introduction

The purpose of the Introduction is to stimulate the reader's interest and to provide background information which is pertinent to the study. The statement of the research question is the most important part of the Introduction. The review of the literature is highly condensed to the most critical and important papers on the topic: a discerning reader or reviewer will be able to identify if the critical papers have been cited. The literature review for a journal manuscript differs strikingly from that for a thesis, in which a detailed review of the literature is mandatory. The content of the Introduction is outlined in Key Points 18.2.

Methods

This section is a description of the study and the outline for the Methods should be taken from the corresponding section of the research proposal (see Chapter 5, p. 31–35). The main consideration is to ensure that enough detail is provided to veri-

fy the findings and to enable replication of the study by an appropriately trained person. Information should be presented in chronological order using the past tense. Subheadings should be used where appropriate, depending on the style of the journal. As an alternative to describing a lengthy procedure, reference may be made to a published paper. Mention of relevant ethics committee'(s)' approval for the study, and that subjects gave informed consent, should be included in the Methods. An outline for the content of the Methods section is provided in Key Points 18.3.

The Methods in a journal manuscript differs from that for a thesis principally in the level of detail provided. Some examples of how the respective sections may differ include:

1. If subjects were recruited in response to advertisements copies of such advertisements

Key Points 18.3

Methods

Contents

Study design	Outline of the study design
Subjects/ Participants	Method of sampling and recruitment, number of subjects and justification of sample size, inclusion, exclusion and withdrawal criteria, method of allocation to study groups, may include descriptive data such as age, gender, body weight
Variables	Independent, dependent, extraneous, controlled
Pilot studies	Outcome of any pilot studies which led to modifications to the main study
Materials	Equipment, instruments or measurement tools (include model number and manufacturer)
Procedures	Detailed description, in chronological order, of exactly what was done and by whom
	Steps taken to ensure reliability and validity and to avoid researcher bias
	Qualitative studies should include methods used to ensure scientific rigour of the data, for example memos, field notes, field observations, interviews, triangulation
Ethical considerations	Major ethical considerations only
Data management/ analyses	Method of calculating derived variables, dealing with outlying values and missing data
	Methods used to summarize data (present tense)
	Computer software (name, version or release number), statistical tests (including a reference for less commonly used tests) and what was compared, critical α probability value at which differences/relationships were considered to be statistically significant

are not included in a journal article, whereas they should appear in the appendices to a thesis.

2. Space limitations in journals allow only a limited number of figures showing procedural set-ups, whereas there is space within a thesis to include figures of all procedural set-ups.

3. Any calibration data and reliability data can only be summarized in a journal article, but should be given in full in a thesis.

4. Pilot studies and their outcomes are often only described in brief in a journal article, whereas a detailed account should be given in a thesis.

Results

The two functions of this section are to report the results (past tense) of the procedures described in the Methods and to present the evidence, i.e. the data (in the form of text, tables or figures), that supports the results. Some journals combine the Results and Discussion into one section (this is often the case when reporting qualitative data from narrative analysis, in which case the section may be headed 'Findings').

There is sometimes confusion as to the difference between results and data: these are defined in Chapter 14 (p. 101).

The content of the Results should be organized to correspond with the order used in the Methods. Alternatively, the most important results should be given first. For example, if a chronological sequence of procedures is described in the Methods then the same order should be used in the Results. If this means that results which answer the question appear late in the Results section, ordering from most to least important should be adopted, thereby giving the answer(s) to the question(s) early on. The order of most to least important should be followed within each paragraph. For every result there must be a method in the Methods. Careful planning of the text, figures and tables is important to ensure that the sequencing of these tells a story.

Before writing the first draft of the Results, it is

important to plan which results are important in answering the question(s) and which can be left out. Only those results which are relevant to the question(s) posed in the Introduction should be included. After deciding which results to present, attention should turn to determining whether data are best presented within the text or as tables or figures. Figures and tables are often used to present details, whereas the narrative section of the Results tends to be used to present the general findings. Clear figures and tables are a very powerful visual means of presenting data and should be used to complement the text, but at the same time must be able to be understood in isolation (see Chapter 15). Except on a few rare occasions, when emphasis is required, data that are given in a table or figure must not be repeated within the text; however, the text can be used to interpret data presented in another form. Most journals require authors to indicate in the text where figures and tables should be placed (this should be close to the related text), but the actual figures and tables should be submitted separately with the manuscript. Photographs of subjects are often placed within the Methods, and should only be used if written informed consent was obtained prior to taking the photograph (see Appendix B). To preserve anonymity, facial features should be covered. If a manuscript includes a figure or table that has already been published, written permission must be obtained from the copyright holder (usually the publisher) and the source acknowledged.

The Results differs in a journal manuscript from that in a thesis because of the space limitations. For example, in a study comparing two groups of subjects it is usual, in a manuscript, to give only group data, whereas in a thesis the data for individual subjects may be included in an appendix. In a manuscript, the reporting of a statistical analysis is usually limited to the test statistic together with the degrees of freedom (e.g. $F_{(1,3)}$) and the P value, whereas it is more common in a thesis to provide the full statistical calculations (e.g. an abbreviated form of the computer printout of the calculations). The reporting of statistics, probability values and the use of the terms 'statistically significant' and 'clinically significant' are covered in Chapter 14 (p. 101).

The Results should not include a discussion of the findings and citations of references, except on the rare occasions when a comparison of raw data with the findings of a published study does not fit well within the Discussion.

Discussion

The purpose of the Discussion is to answer the question(s) posed in the Introduction, explain how the results support the answers and how the answers fit in with existing knowledge of the topic. The Discussion should be considered the heart of the paper, and invariably requires several attempts at writing. This is the main section in which the author can express their interpretations and opinions, for example how important they think the results are, their suggestions for future research and the implications of the findings. In order to make the message clear, the Discussion should be kept as short as possible while still clearly and fully stating, supporting, explaining and defending the answers to the questions as well as discussing other important and directly relevant issues. Side issues and unnecessary issues should not be included as these tend to obscure the message. Care must be taken to provide a commentary and not a reiteration of the Results. The recommended content of the Discussion is given in Key Points 18.4.

The organization of the content is important. The Discussion should begin by stating answer(s) to the question(s) and supporting the answer(s) with the results. It should not begin with a summary of the results or indications for further research, or recommendations for changes in clinical practice. At the end of the Discussion the answer(s) should be restated and an indication of the importance of the research provided by stating applications, implications or speculations. Again, owing to space limitations, the Discussion in a journal manuscript is much shorter than that in a thesis.

The question(s) should be answered using the same key terms and the same verbs (present tense) that were used when posing the question(s) in the Introduction. The answer must be

Key Points 18.4

Discussion

Contents

Answers	Answer(s) to the question(s) posed in the Introduction together with accompanying support and defence of the answers by reference to published studies
Explanations of	How the findings concur with those of others
	Any discrepancies of the results with those of others
	Unexpected findings
Indications of	The limitations of the study which may affect the study validity or generalizability of the study findings
	Any results that do not support the answers
	The originality/uniqueness of the work
	The importance of the work, for example, its clinical significance
Recommendations for	Further research
	Changes in clinical practice (where appropriate)

confined to the population studied: for example, if the subjects were randomly selected from a population with osteoarthritis of the knee, the findings can only be generalized to the population with osteoarthritis of the knee and not to a population with knee pain from other causes. If more than one question was asked in the Introduction, they must all be answered in the Discussion. All results relating to the question should be addressed, irrespective of whether or not the findings were statistically significant. Answers to questions that were never asked must not be included.

The answer(s) should be supported whenever possible by reference to published work. It may be necessary to explain an answer by saying why

it is acceptable and how it is consistent or fits in with published ideas on the topic. When defending an answer it is necessary to explain why it is more satisfactory than other answers, and why those other answers are unsatisfactory. Where the findings of the study are not in agreement with those of others, this discrepancy should be explained. The sequencing of this information is important: the results of the present study should be discussed before citing the work of others. In the event that unexpected findings occur, a decision should be made as to whether these are of little importance or may be very exciting. Demonstrating a willingness to discuss and evaluate rival explanations for the results is the hallmark of a good Discussion. When discussing an unexpected finding, the sentence should begin by saying it was unexpected, followed by the best possible explanation.

Weaknesses in study design, for example extraneous variables that only became apparent during the conduct of the study, should be discussed. The relative importance of these limitations to the interpretation of the results and how they may affect the validity or the generalizability of the findings requires comment. When identifying the limitations an apologetic tone should be avoided and the study accepted for what it is. If an author identifies fundamental limitations of the study the reader may question why it was undertaken.

A concise summary of the principal implications of the findings should be given and, regardless of statistical significance, the clinical importance (where appropriate) of the findings addressed. Based on the findings, where appropriate, recommendations for clinical practice should be made. When discussing the implications, verbs that suggest some uncertainty, such as 'suggest', 'imply' or 'speculate', should be used. As all research leads to further questions, recommendations for further research should be given, but the temptation to provide a long list should be avoided and one or two major recommendations focused on. Suggestions for further research should not include those which could have been easily addressed within the study, as this shows there has been inadequate planning, examination or interpretation of the data.

Conclusions

This section should comprise a brief statement of the major findings and implications of the study. It is not the function of this section to summarize the study: this is the purpose of the Abstract. New information must not be included in the Conclusions.

References

References are almost exclusively used in the Introduction and the Discussion. The references should be the most valid and the most available (see Chapter 14, p. 106).

The 'Guidelines for Authors' will invariably state the reference system to be used; if not, recent issues of the journal should be carefully examined and the required referencing system followed meticulously.

Acknowledgements

All important contributors should be acknowledged, for example persons who provided statistical or technical advice and assistance, the subjects, those who helped with recruitment, and personnel who helped with the preparation of the manuscript (see Chapter 16, p. 129). If the research was supported by a grant, the name of the funding body must be included.

PRIOR TO MANUSCRIPT SUBMISSION

It is recommended that authors conduct a 'mock review' prior to manuscript submission. This is an invaluable process as it allows for scrutiny of the manuscript by others who have not been involved in its preparation.

The ideal scenario is to select two or three colleagues who are familiar with the topic and who have a record of publication. If such persons are not available it is still important and useful to undertake a review. When possible, three colleagues should be asked to review the manuscript or portions of it. Ideally there should be one person who is familiar with the topic, one who is representative of the readership of the journal to which the manuscript is being submitted, and a third person who has experience in writing for publication. In addition, and where possible, it may help to ask a statistician to review part of the manuscript. When seeking constructive criticism, it is important to clarify for each colleague which sections of the manuscript they are being asked to address. Once the manuscript has been revised to take account of the comments received, it is useful to ask the same persons for their comments on the revision. The final step prior to submission is to proofread the manuscript (see Chapter 14, p. 107–108).

MANUSCRIPT SUBMISSION

The manuscript should now be ready for submission. The original and the required number of copies should be sent with a covering letter to the editor of the chosen journal. Although most photocopier reproduction is of a high standard, it is recommended that the original copy is marked 'original' (in pencil) in the top right-hand corner of the title page. The submitted manuscript will include the following:

- Preliminary pages – title page with author details and key words
- Sections of the manuscript – Abstract, Introduction, Methods, Results, Discussion, Conclusions, Acknowledgements, References
- Attachments – copies of any figures or tables.

It is usually mandatory to include with the manuscript a copyright release statement signed by all authors at the time of submission, or upon acceptance of the manuscript. Details of the content of this statement may be provided in the 'Guidelines for Authors' or will be sent by the editor with the letter of acceptance. Some journals also require an electronic copy of the manuscript, either at the time of submission or when a manuscript has been accepted for publication.

The covering letter which accompanies the manuscript should be addressed to the appropriate editor of the journal. Some professional journals have both a 'managing' editor and a scientific editor; the scientific editor is responsible for overseeing the review process. An example of a suitable covering letter is given below:

Dear Dr Smith,

Please find enclosed the original and three copies of our manuscript entitled 'Speech therapy in the management of dysphagia: results of a controlled trial' which we would like to have considered for publication in the International Journal of Speech Pathology. Please could you acknowledge receipt of this manuscript.

Authors should include in the covering letter a brief statement saying why the topic of the manuscript is important (i.e. arguing the key original features) and why it will be of interest to the readers of the journal. Although it is usual practice to acknowledge receipt of a manuscript, it is still wise to request this in order to confirm that the manuscript reached its destination. The editor will respond to this request and, in doing so, will provide a manuscript reference number for use in all subsequent correspondence.

Authors should assume that the review process will take a minimum of 3–4 months. This includes the time needed for preliminary screening of the manuscript by the editor (assistant editors or members of the editorial board), distribution to the reviewers, the period allocated to the reviewers to provide their comments (often between 4 and 8 weeks), correspondence between the reviewers and the editor and the return of the manuscript to the author(s). If an excessively long time elapses between submission and receipt of the reviewers' comments it is reasonable to send a polite letter to the editor inquiring as to when a response might be expected.

THE REVIEW PROCESS

The review process will vary slightly from one journal to another. It commonly begins with in-house screening of the manuscript by the editor, associate editor(s) or one or more members of the editorial board. Manuscripts which are considered to be of an acceptable standard and present research on topics consistent with the focus of the journal are sent to two or three external reviewers, together with guidelines for the review process.

Manuscripts which do not satisfy these criteria are returned to the author(s) with a covering letter outlining the reasons for rejection. Reviewers are usually selected on the basis of possessing adequate knowledge of the topic of the research as well as a track record in publication. Many journals publish a list of the names of the external reviewers in each issue of the journal, or in one issue each year. Some journals may also seek the opinion of a statistician. Reviewers are generally allowed 4–8 weeks to complete their review. Upon receipt of the reviewers' comments the editor, associate editor(s) or members of the editorial board review the manuscript and a decision is made whether to accept it for publication. Acceptance is almost invariably subject to further revision, and often a re-review (Henderson 1995).

Authors need to be prepared for the possibility of a long time elapsing between submitting the manuscript and receiving feedback. For successful manuscripts there is a further delay between final acceptance and publication. Some journals publish the dates when the manuscript was first received and the date of acceptance (often 1–3 years later): this provides the intending author with an idea of the expected time lag.

AUTHOR'S RESPONSES TO THE EDITOR

It is unusual for a manuscript to be accepted without any changes being required; however, if this is the case it is polite to respond to the editor:

Dear Dr Smith,

Re: MS 242 Speech therapy in the management of dysphagia: results of a controlled trial

Thank you for your letter dated 20th January 1998. We are pleased that the manuscript has been accepted for publication in the journal and look forward to receiving the proofs in due course.

At this time it may also be necessary to send an electronic copy of the manuscript and a signed copyright release statement, if not already submitted. The electronic copy will be used during preparation of the manuscript for printing. Close to the time of publication (often 2–4 weeks prior to publication) the author who has been named for all correspondence will receive a copy of the proofs for checking. Often only 1–2 days are allowed for this task, which requires prompt action and 100% attention to detail. Particular attention should be paid to figures and tables, as the publisher may have had to reformat or resize these to fit the journal layout. This is the last chance to ensure that the published manuscript is an accurate replica of the one accepted. Proofs are only for checking and not for rewriting: changes in the text at this stage will be very expensive. If an important mistake is noted (due to error on the part of the author) the editor of the journal should be contacted.

There will be occasions when a manuscript is rejected by a journal. Although at the time this may seem devastating, rejection does not necessarily imply that the manuscript will not be published elsewhere. The contents of the editor's letter and the comments of the reviewers must be carefully examined. The manuscript may be rejected because the reviewers consider it necessary to gather more data (e.g. the studying of additional subjects in an attempt to improve the statistical power of the study) or perform further analysis. Other reasons may be that the topic is unsuitable for the journal, or because major restructuring of the manuscript is necessary. Irrespective of the reasons for rejection, it is wise to consider the comments carefully and revise the manuscript before submission to an alternative journal. There may be occasions when the author(s) dispute the decision to reject the manuscript on the grounds that it appears from the reviewers' comments there has been some misunderstanding, or the comments suggest a lack of knowledge in the subject area. In such cases it is reasonable to write to the editor asking whether he or she will reconsider the decision. In making such a request it is essential for the author(s) to justify why there are major concerns with the reviewers' comments. The chance of having the decision reconsidered is more likely when the different reviewers disagree on important points. However, such a request must be not be made lightly as the editor will have selected the reviewers because of their experience in research and the assumption that they possess the relevant experience to provide a critique of the manuscript.

Although some manuscripts are accepted or rejected immediately, it is most common for a manuscript to be 'accepted' subject to specific changes being made. The following section discusses strategies for responding to comments raised by the reviewers in the case of a manuscript which requires revision and resubmission. Other examples of responses to a reviewer's comments can be found in Chapter 17 (p. 144–145).

Reviewers will differ in their manner and the level of detail provided in their comments. In addition to comments relating to the content of the manuscript, some reviewers will suggest changes in wording and will identify any typographical, grammatical or spelling errors, or errors in the references which were missed during proofreading. The author(s) should respond separately to the comments of each reviewer and, in doing so, answer all the criticisms raised. Responses should make clear how the reviewers' recommendations have been incorporated into the revised manuscript, together with a cross-reference to the relevant page(s) and paragraph(s). This approach reduces the workload for the editor and reviewers by eliminating the necessity to search through the entire manuscript to find the changes. The following is an example of a response to a comment raised:

The authors agree that the inclusion of data relating to the subjects' past medical histories and episodes of hospitalization would be a useful addition to the manuscript. This information has been included in the Results (page 6, para 2) of the revised manuscript.

The author(s) may disagree with some of the comments or be unable to follow the recommendations suggested. In this case it is necessary to explain why changes have not been made and, where appropriate, support the explanation with reference to relevant literature. For example:

Although we accept that it would have been useful to study the subjects in the immediate period following discharge from hospital, 15 of the subjects (i.e. 75%) did not live in the metropolitan area and thus it was not feasible to study these subjects as outpatients. A comment to this effect has been included in the Discussion (page 10, para 4). In addition, the findings of the study by Allen and Jones (1994), who conducted a 3-month follow-up of 142 subjects following discharge from hospital, showed only minimal improvement in function following cessation of physiotherapy. Reference to this point has been made in the Discussion (page 12, para 3).

The author(s) should not compromise scientific integrity when responding to the reviewers' comments and making changes to the manuscript; however, it may be reasonable to agree to small changes which are of lesser importance. When each point has been addressed and the revised manuscript and responses to the reviewers carefully proofread, the required number of copies of the manuscript should be submitted with a covering letter to the editor. The covering letter should begin with a statement thanking the editor and the reviewers for their interest in the manuscript and for the comments provided. This demonstrates that the author(s) value the time taken by the reviewers to undertake this task. If only minimal revision is necessary the editor may accept the revisions without seeking comment from the original reviewers. For major revisions it is usual to resubmit the manuscript to the original reviewers and, on occasions, to new reviewers.

In summary, the preparation of a manuscript which is accepted for publication in a journal is a challenging and worthwhile experience. This should be associated with a sense of achievement and pride on the part of the author(s).

REFERENCES

Henderson K 1995 Careful manuscript preparation maximizes publication potential. Australian Journal of Physiotherapy 41(4): 237–240

Further Reading

American Psychological Association 1994 Publication manual of the American Psychological Association, 4th edn. American Psychological Association, Washington

Bork C E 1993 Research in physical therapy. Lippincott, Philadelphia

Currier D P 1990 Elements in physical therapy, 3rd edn. Williams & Wilkins, Baltimore

DePoy E, Gitlin L N 1994 Introduction to research. Mosby, St. Louis

Jenkins S 1995 How to write a paper for a scientific journal. Australian Journal of Physiotherapy 41(4): 285–290

Lister M J 1989 Writing manuscripts for a scientific journal. Physiotherapy Theory and Practice 5: 147–155

Morse J M, Field P A 1995 Qualitative research methods for health professionals, 2nd edn. Sage Publications, Thousand Oaks

Portney L G, Watkins M P 1993 Foundations of clinical research. Applications to practice. Appleton and Lange, Connecticut, pp. 583–599

Rudestam K E, Newton R R 1992 Surviving your dissertation. Sage Publications, Newbury Park

Zeiger M 1991 Essentials of writing biomedical research papers. McGraw-Hill, New York

Presenting research

Verbal presentations are an important method of communicating research ideas, proposals and findings. Typical situations for research presentations include presenting a paper at a scientific conference, presenting a research seminar to a university or hospital department or special interest group, and presenting as part of academic studies. The researching therapist may also be required to present to a funding organization or to the wider community.

Good verbal communication skills are essential for every professional and the ability to present research is particularly important. Effective presentations are useful as they enable information to be communicated. For example, a presentation to a special interest group seminar may inform members of that group about some issue which is important to their practice. Another reason presentations are important is because they are used to judge the knowledge, authority and competence of the presenter. Thus a professional is likely to lose the respect of their peers, and patients, if they present poorly on a number of occasions.

Very few people are naturally good at presenting a paper verbally, and most presenters are anxious and nervous about presenting. However, with good preparation it should be possible for nearly anyone to give a good verbal presentation.

This chapter outlines how to prepare the content and audiovisual (AV) aids for a presentation, how to deliver a presentation and how to deal with question time.

Hazard 19.1

Nearly everyone has suffered through a poor presentation. Typical reasons for presentations not being effective include:

Thinking a written paper can be simply read out loud as a verbal presentation

Poor content

Poor organization of content

Poor presentation of content

Too many slides

Poor/too detailed slides

Poor time management

Poor verbal skills

PREPARATION

Preparing for a successful presentation is a lengthy process and involves the preparation of the scientific content and the AV aids as well as choosing the speaking style to adopt. However, before this can take place some background information is needed.

Background information

Typically, background information which the researching therapist should acquire includes: who will be the audience, what type of presentation is expected, what is the purpose of the presentation, how long are the presentation and discussion times and what is the venue of the presentation?

Audience

Perhaps the single most important aspect of background information in terms of how it will guide the preparation and delivery of a presentation is the determination of the characteristics of the anticipated audience. Typically, audiences may include peers, professionals from other specialty areas and non-professionals. The content, style and language of the presentation will clearly need to be modified to suit the audience. This is crucial, as an audience may feel insulted if the level of language is too simple, yet will not be informed nor convinced if they do not understand the presentation (e.g. if too much technical jargon is used).

Type of presentation

After consideration of the expected audience and how this will constrain various aspects of the presentation, the type of presentation should be considered. There are a number of different types of research presentation, and each has its special requirements. Common types include conference papers, research proposal presentations and departmental seminars. The type of presentation tends to set the style, for example how formal the presentation will be. The details provided in this chapter are aimed at a conference presentation, although most are applicable to all types of presentations.

Purpose of presentation

To some extent the purpose of the presentation will be determined by the type: for example, when presenting at a scientific conference a typical purpose would be to inform an audience about research that had been performed. Similarly, presenting a research proposal would have the purpose of providing peers, supervisors, etc. with the opportunity to review a proposed study, and a presentation to a clinical group may have the purpose of encouraging colleagues to change aspects of their practice. Another purpose for a presentation is to provide information to form the basis of a discussion with colleagues, commonly called a seminar. Whatever the purpose is, it should be kept in mind throughout the preparation of a presentation and used to evaluate it during practice sessions.

Length of presentation

The audience, type and purpose of a presentation are vital aspects affecting its content and style. However, content is often limited by the time available: in most instances the length of a presentation is set by the organizers of the event. Conference papers are typically 10–20 minutes in length, followed by 5–10 minutes of questions and discussion. The time available for higher degree research proposal presentations and discussion varies considerably, from 10–20 minutes to an almost open-ended discussion lasting several hours. Talks to special interest groups and departmental seminars are typically less than 1 hour. Whatever the overall time available, it is usually important to allow sufficient time for discussion following a presentation. Sometimes the length of discussion time is also specified by the event organizers. When this has not been specified, it is important to consider the audience and the purpose of the presentation, and to plan sufficient discussion time.

Venue

The size of the venue, and hence probably the audience, is also important to consider in the planning stages. Large venues usually need a more formal presentation and a high quality of AV aids is essential. Presentations in large venues usually require the use of more technology, for example a microphone and perhaps a laser pointer. Venues will also have a 'feel' which, along with size, will influence the interaction between presenter and audience. Other technical aspects of a venue to consider are the arrangement of seating and the control of the lighting, as these will influence the visual aspects of a presentation and the optimal design of AV aids.

Specific requirements

Finally, a presenter needs to know whether the organizers of an event have stipulated certain requirements. For example, the projection facilities may be limited to overhead transparencies (OHTs), or the only type of microphone available may be fixed to a lectern, thus restricting the movement of the presenter. With international conferences it is also important to note the language to be spoken during the presentations.

Content

Structure

Once the background to the presentation has been established, planning of the content can begin. The first phase is laying out the structure of the presentation. One of the aspects that makes research presentations easier than an after-dinner speech is that there is a strong convention for structure: introduction, body, conclusion. It is wise to follow this convention. The following is written specifically for a 10-minute conference presentation, although the information is applicable to most presentations.

Title

The title should provide a clear and succinct description of the presentation. The formality of the title depends on the type of presentation. For a paper in a scientific session of a major conference the title should probably be formal and scientific, whereas for a local special interest group seminar it may be appropriate to have a more colloquial title. Examples of titles for two presentations on the same research, but to different audiences, illustrate this:

An ethnographic evaluation of the physician–therapist–client triad

Do therapists hear what clients say?

Introduction

The first section of a presentation is the Introduction. The first few minutes of a verbal presentation are vital: if the essential information is not presented, or is presented in an inappropriate way, the attention of the audience will be lost. Four elements need to be covered in the Introduction: the problem, its significance, a brief critical review of the most important literature, and the aim of the research. This information should be presented confidently to encourage the audience to settle quickly. The introduction should take 2–3 minutes.

Body

The second section is the body of the presentation, and is where the substance of the research is presented. Elements covered typically include methods, results and discussion.

In conference presentations an overview of the methods is normally all that is required, as the details are provided in the written proceedings if available. Sometimes a single diagram or photograph is the clearest way of communicating an overview of the methods. Usually only two to four key results should be presented in a short presentation. This will allow an adequate description of the results and an adequate discussion. Where possible, figures should be used to present the key results. The discussion should include an explanation of the results and the implications of the key results. Often it is easier for an audience to follow if the discussion specific to particular results is presented before the next key result. The body of the presentation should take 6–7 minutes.

Conclusion

The final section is the conclusion, which should encapsulate the important aspects of the presentation. It should include a summary of the aim of the research and the key results, conclusions drawn from the results, and their implications. This provides a concise 'take home' message for the audience. The conclusion should take 1–2 minutes.

Moulding the information

When all the content is collated the order should be reviewed to ensure a logical sequence. The content should be carefully edited to delete any non-essential information. The aim of a good presentation is to tell a story, so the information should be arranged to produce a logical flow which takes the audience on a clear path from Introduction to Conclusion. The audience should always be clear about how each bit of information fits into the whole story.

Once the content has been edited to create a clear story, the presenter is nearly ready to prepare the AV aids. A useful method for ensuring that the story is clear, and of determining AV needs, is to prepare the presentation in 'storyboard' form. A storyboard is a series of sketches representing the slides the audience will be seeing, with notes about what will be said under each sketch. Figure 19.1 shows the beginning of a storyboard, with the first two slides and accompanying notes.

The notes prepared for the storyboard can be developed into prompt notes or cue cards, one per slide. These can be used as a memory support during the actual presentation. Some presenters write what they intend to say, word for word (see notes under first slide in Fig. 19.1). During practice sessions the notes are read aloud and edited until the presenter is happy with the words. Having an actual script can prevent a nervous presenter getting stuck for words. However, during the presentation it can be difficult to keep track of progress and the flow of the presentation may be interrupted. To prevent this, key words and phrases can be highlighted on the final version to make it easy to find one's place. The other disadvantage of writing the talk word for word is that one may be tempted to read, rather than present, the information. As this inhibits eye contact and may decrease audience attention, it should only be used as a last resort by a very nervous presenter.

Prompt notes which contain only key words and phrases are preferable (see notes under second slide in Fig. 19.1). With adequate preparation during rehearsals the presenter usually develops confidence in what to say about each point and how to say it, thus requiring only key words to prompt the next thought. An advantage of this approach is that small cards can be used to write the key points and phrases for each slide. (Remember the lights may be dimmed during a presentation, so notes should be written in a large, high-contrast font.) A further advantage is that the presenter will be encouraged to look at and engage the audience.

Once the storyboard has been edited so that the presentation flows well, the AV aids can be prepared.

> A comparison of clinic
> and worksite work
> hardening programmes
>
> R.
> Therapist

> Introduction
>
> * work related back problems
> a major problem
> * high cost of injury
> * affects quality of life
> * legislation in different
> countries supports different
> work hardening approaches

*Good afternoon, the title
of my presentation is...*

*First, I would like to present an
introduction into the importance
of the problem of rehabilitation
of work-related back problems
and discuss how approaches to
rehabilitation are partly
determined by legislation.*

*I will then outline the aim of the
study, its methods and main
findings. In discussing the main
findings I will draw the clinical
implications to your attention.*

*I will be happy to discuss
questions and comments
following my presentation.*

major problem.

*cost to community
rehabilitation costs
  Samson et al 1995 $6,500
Lost work productivity
Delilah 1994 13%.*

*cost to individual
finances, loss of career,
loss of family role,
socialisation.
Jezebel 1995 ...*

*legislation in Australia
early return to limited work
work hardening at worksite
Jonah 1993...*

*legislation in many USA
states does not support early
return to work
clinic based work hardening...
Legislation in Canada, UK,
NZ, SA..*

Figure 19.1   Example of a 'storyboard'

Audiovisual aids

There is a wide range of AV aids from which to choose and the presenter needs to determine which is appropriate and available for a particular presentation. It is important to remember that the role of AV aids is to assist the presenter to convey information to the audience.

The most commonly used aids are a microphone and a projection system. Commonly used visual projection systems include OHTs, 35 mm slides and computer-generated slide shows.

Other AV aids which may be useful include video tape, audio tape, pointers, props and demonstrations. Props are objects used to demonstrate an aspect of the presentation to the audience. For example, a chair and model spine may be used as props to demonstrate to the audience the different options for correct sitting posture. With the increasing availability of technology at venues, the benefits of such demonstrations seem to have been forgotten: some presenters needlessly spend hours taking and editing video tape to present something which they could easily demonstrate 'live' to the audience. An additional benefit of demonstrations is that they are not technology dependent and can therefore be used when no projection facilities are available.

Slides

Most presentations use some form of 'slide', that is, OHTs, 35 mm slides or computer-generated slides. These are a very important part of a presentation, and reflect the presenter's ability to think clearly about a topic and present information clearly and concisely. There are a number of features of slides which are applicable whatever medium is used to project them. The remainder of this section provides a practical guide to the task of designing good slides.

It is important to remember that slides should evolve with the evolution of the spoken part of the presentation. Thus, drafts of the slides should be sketched on sheets of paper (or directly on a computer if a computer slide generator is to be used) and during practice presentations these should be edited so that they are integrated with the spoken text and support the audience's understanding. Only when the presentation has been refined to the extent that it is working effectively and the story is clear, should the actual slides for projection be processed.

Presentations are made more effective when slides reinforce the spoken word, are used in an appropriate number, have good layout and clear elements and make sensible use of colour.

The purpose of slides is to reinforce the spoken word, therefore the visual image needs to be congruent with what the audience is hearing. Once a slide becomes visible the audience will tend to read the whole of it before returning their attention to what is being said. It is therefore preferable for the information on a slide to be concise enough to be read in a few seconds.

Each slide usually requires about a minute of speaking time on average. Some may need less time (e.g. title slide) and some may need a little longer (e.g. graph of results). Thus, a maximum of around 10 slides are commonly needed for a 10-minute presentation. Too few slides will usually

mean there are either blank periods or periods where the spoken word is not addressing the text on the slide. (A scenery slide may be used to fill a period when the display of irrelevant text would distract from the verbal presentation.) Too many slides results in a machine gun-like visual barrage of the audience which is likely to hinder communication and understanding. Some presentations benefit from dual slide projection, particularly if one slide consistently presents photographs or graphics while salient points are shown on the other. However, as with all systems, the more elements that are added, the more likely the system is to fail!

 Hazard 19.2

Common mistakes with slides:

Talking about something when a slide on another issue is on display

Too many slides

Too much detail on each slide

Not enough detail on slide (e.g. Subjects – inclusion, exclusion, withdrawal criteria)

In terms of their general layout slides need to be clear and uncluttered. The important part needs to be near the centre of the slide as image quality and visibility often deteriorate near the edges. Slide backgrounds and text and graphic elements need to complement each other. For 35 mm slides it is important to try to keep all the presentation in the same format, either horizontal (landscape) or vertical (portrait). Landscape is preferable, as the audience may not be able to see the bottom half of portrait-orientated slides in many venues.

The background for slides needs to be simple and of consistent lightness or darkness. The use of borders and fancy frames should be kept to a minimum as these can detract from, and reduce the space available for, useful information. With computer-generated slides it is preferable to avoid the temptation to use lots of extraneous graphics, such as multiple borders and dramatic background patterns. Backgrounds which graduate from light to dark should only be used if the lightest part of background is substantially darker than the text, to maintain high contrast.

Text on slides should be minimal. It is not necessary to write in full sentences – in fact, point form is preferable. After initial planning, draft slides should be edited carefully to remove redundant words. Common abbreviations are acceptable and help keep slides uncluttered. Punctuation is usually unnecessary and should be removed.

For slides to be easy for the audience to read there needs to be high contrast between the text and the background and the text needs to be sufficiently large and clear. To ensure high contrast, black (or dark) text on a clear background should be used for OHTs and a white (or very light) text on a dark background for 35 mm and computer-generated slides. Font sizes 18–36 pt for the text body and 36–60 pt for headings will ensure that the text is large enough. Sans serif fonts (Helvetica, Arial) generally provide better text to background contrast and produce a clearer image when projected. All capitals should be avoided (see Appendix E). Figure 19.2 shows an example of a poor slide and Figure 19.3 is an example of a good slide.

Graphic elements on slides provide an excellent opportunity for presenters to help the audience see what they are talking about. Graphics commonly used in presentations are graphs and photographs. Flow charts may also be used to describe a study design efficiently.

Graphs are an excellent way of demonstrating important aspects of the results being presented. Graphs should be simple, with a concise title and axes labelled (including units). It is preferable to have only two to four data groups displayed on any one graph (Chapter 15 provides details on the preparation of figures and tables). When a

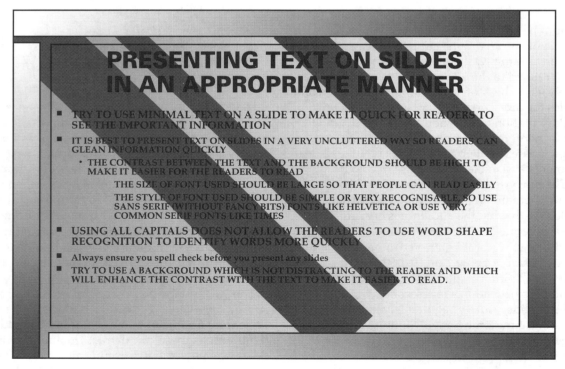

Figure 19.2 Example of a poor text slide. (Note: clutter, poor contrast, busy background, use of all capitals, too much text, spelling errors)

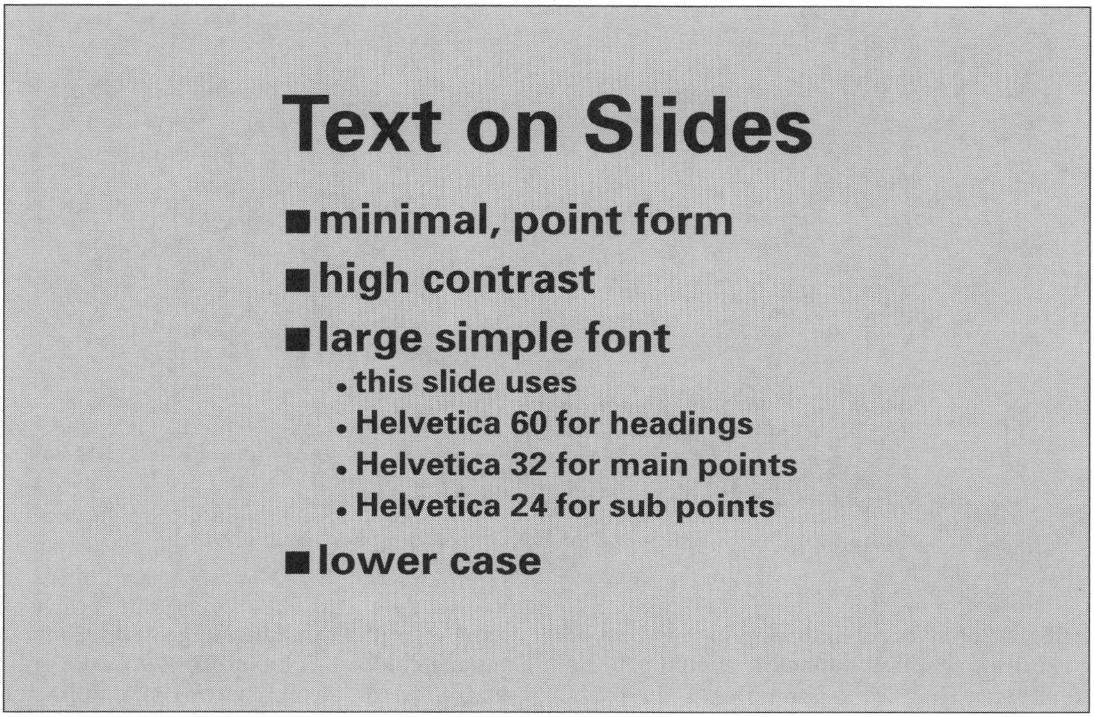

Figure 19.3   Example of a good text slide

graph is first presented to an audience it should be introduced, that is, the audience should be told what the axes are and what the data are (for example individual data or group mean and standard deviation data) before they are told about the important trends, etc. This description also allows the audience time to assimilate the graph. An example of such a description follows.

This figure shows a histogram of the number of speech therapists working in schools. On the x axis are the different States of Australia and on the y axis is the total number of speech therapists for each State. You will notice that Western Australia has an unusually large number of speech therapists in schools compared with the other States.

Photographs enable considerable detail to be conveyed to the audience very quickly. They are particularly useful for describing complex spatial information such as an experimental set-up or posture (Fig. 19.4). However, only good-quality photographs should be used: they need to have sharp focus and be correctly exposed and should not contain distracting irrelevant detail (e.g. other equipment in the background or a fussy backdrop). The identity of people shown in any photographs may need to be hidden and their permission should be obtained before the photographs are shown (see Appendix B).

Tables are sometimes used but are often better left to the written report, because it usually takes more time to understand the data presented and any pattern in the data. Presentations should focus on summaries of the data or patterns, which can usually be better represented in graphs. However, if data are clearly summarized and key points emphasized visually, tables can be used. Any table used in a presentation should be simple, preferably with only four or six cells. Font sizes similar to those suggested for main points (32 pt) and sub-points (24 pt) should be used.

Colour is an important component of human vision and therefore needs to be used carefully. Eight percent of males and 0.4% of females have

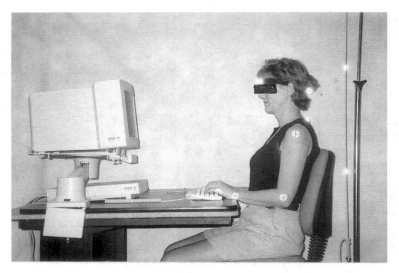

Figure 19.4   Example of a clear photograph of an experimental set-up

some degree of colour blindness, so it is best to design slides so contrasts are clear even if colours are removed. That is, lightness and darkness should be used as the primary contrast and colour should only be used as secondary contrast.

Light colours on a dark background have a very strong attention-grabbing effect. For 35 mm and computer-generated slides it is therefore wise to use background colours which are definitely dark, preferably black or blue. Foreground detail such as text should therefore be light, preferably white or perhaps yellow. When using OHTs black text on a clear background provides the best contrast, although a dark colour on very light or clear background is acceptable. When colour is used for text or detail in figures on OHTs the colour should be dark enough to provide adequate contrast with the light background.

To be effective colour needs to be used sparingly to avoid the 'Christmas tree' look. Sensible use enables colour to assist the clarity of the visual image. For example, if the presenter wishes to highlight the grouping of multiple items this can be achieved by using the very strong grouping effect of the same colour. Alternatively, if the presenter wishes to highlight differences between items a contrast can be suggested by using contrasting colours. For example, within a graph the separation of elements can be emphasized by using contrasting colours (e.g. red and green, or blue and yellow). Likewise, to emphasize similarity similar colours should be used (such as orange and yellow, blue and violet). When three to four elements are presented in a figure, red, yellow, green, blue and white make good distinct colours, although orange, yellow-green, blue-green and violet are acceptable. (Extra care should be taken when using red on blue, as some people will have difficulty with this combination since they are at the opposite ends of the visual spectrum.)

Use of audiovisual aids

A presenter needs to be competent in the use of AV aids. Competence and confidence come with practice, therefore it is important to be familiar with the AV equipment proposed for a presentation. If possible the AV aids should be tested in the actual presentation room. If this is not possible a venue where the lighting, distances etc. are similar can be used. The presenter should practise integrating the AV aids into the presentation and modify them and/or the spoken word to ensure a cohesive and clear story. Prior to the start of a presentation, and preferably before the audience has arrived, a presenter should become familiar with the operation of any AV equipment to be used. A good presenter will also plan what to do if equipment fails. For example, they may need to quickly sketch graphs showing the results on a whiteboard, or demonstrate some aspect of subject behaviour if the slide projection system fails. This is particularly important when using computer-generated graphs. (The possession of notes or prompt cards in addition to the slides also enables the presenter to continue if the projection system fails.)

Although they are not strictly considered an AV aid, lecterns are another piece of equipment that the presenter must contend with. Unfortunately, lecterns are often designed to be suitable for males of average height. Thus, half of the male presenters and around 95% of female presenters will find the lectern too high, and half the male presenters and a smaller proportion of female presenters will find it too low. For shorter individuals this problem can be overcome by standing on a platform behind the lectern. Lecterns provide a holder for prompt notes, give the presenter something secure to hold on to if they are feeling a little shaky, and help to hide the odd postures and movements of some speakers' legs. If the lectern has a built-in light and microphone, the presenter should practise with these, with someone in the audience to give feedback on the visual and auditory effects.

If a microphone is to be used it is important to consider the following points. Most microphones are direction and distance sensitive. This means that if a presenter varies the distance from their mouth to the microphone, or the direction of their head, the audience will hear variations in voice volume. Voice volume is an important part of a presentation and should be consciously used. A random fluctuation of volume is distracting for the audience. If a fixed microphone is being used it is important that the presenter moves only within an arc around it, always remaining a fixed distance away. The voice should be directed so that it goes over the top of the microphone. If a presenter needs to move around, or if they are unable to control their movements during a presentation, a mobile microphone should be used. Often called a lapel microphone, mobile microphones are small and should be attached to the presenter about 10 cm below the larynx. (Care should be taken to select clothing with a lapel or similar.) Mobile microphones may be attached to the amplifier by a long lead (in which case beware of the trip hazard) or may be attached by a short lead to a radio transmitter (about the size of a small radio) which is worn by the presenter.

When using slides or OHTs, as each slide is presented the presenter should glance to check that it is the correct slide and is positioned correctly (particularly for OHTs). Having a small reproduction of the slide on a prompt card will make this easier. The presenter should take care to turn back to face the audience before beginning to speak: they should not speak to the screen.

A pointer may be used to emphasize key points on the slide and is especially useful to highlight trends on graphs. However, the use of a pointer can be distracting and can highlight the presenter's nervousness. When pointing to 35 mm or computer slide images a stick or wand may be used in a well-lit room, whereas a laser or light pointer may be used in a darkened room. As the pointer will magnify a shaking hand, bracing the pointer or hand on the lectern or on the other elbow will help. For pointing to OHTs a pen or similar object on the projector itself may be used, rather than pointing to the screen and thus turning away from the audience.

DELIVERY

Once the presentation has been prepared and the AV equipment arranged, the presenter should be ready. Critical aspects of the delivery are the use of voice and body, the management of performance anxiety and the conduct of question time.

Voice

Good presentations depend on a clear, crisp voice of appropriate pace, volume and intonation. Most presenters tend to speak too rapidly when nervous, and will therefore need to speak at a pace which feels slightly slow. Similarly, many presenters tend to speak too quietly, resulting in the volume being insufficient. Volume should also be used, within a limited range, to add variety to a presentation. Thus important points can be emphasized by increasing the volume slightly. Voice intonation is also important. To keep and maintain audience interest the presenter's voice should be lively and enthusiastic, though appropriate to the formality of the occasion. Intonation can also be used to distinguish between a main point and a subsidiary point. Finally, voice pitch needs to be controlled. People often speak with a higher pitch when nervous, so to imply confidence and calmness a presenter should try to speak in a slightly lower pitch than their normal voice. A rising intonation at the end of each sentence suggests insecurity and should be reserved for questions.

Body

Good presenters use eye contact to engage the audience, and should look at the audience and not at the screen when talking. Good presenters look at all parts of the audience to give all members the impression they are being spoken to directly. However, they should avoid continually looking directly at one place or person. Good presenters also tend to smile: this helps to relax the speaker and engage the audience. Body posture should be erect but relaxed, to imply confidence.

Body movements are important to add animation and to express enthusiasm, but presenters should avoid repetitive movements indicative of nervousness, such as fiddling (with a pen, slide pointer, hair, clothes, rings), hand wringing, head bobbing or rocking back and forth or side to side. If nervous fiddling cannot be controlled the hands should be kept in the pockets, and keys and coins removed so that the noise is reduced.

A presenter needs to plan where to position their body, taking care not to block the audience's view. If a lectern with fixed microphone is being used the presenter is restricted in their movement. If a lapel microphone, or no microphone, is being used the presenter may wish to move around, but must be careful not to appear like a psychologically disturbed wild animal pacing up and down its cage!

Practice

Rehearsal of a presentation is essential. Some mental rehearsal is useful in the early stages of preparation. When the presentation appears to be ready, a presenter should perform several practice deliveries, speaking out loud and using the AV aids. An excellent way to get feedback on the practice presentation is to invite colleagues (and the supervisor) who are likely to give some honest, constructive criticism. Another useful technique is to record the practice delivery on audio or video tape, preferably the latter, to enable self-criticism.

Presenters should anticipate problems and practise dealing with them (e.g. projector failure mid presentation). This is particularly important for presentations using computer-generated slides as computer failure may leave the presenter with only a disk in hand.

On the day

On the day the presentation is due a check should be conducted to ensure that the prompt cards/notes are available and that the presentation aids are functioning. The presenter should plan to arrive at the venue well in advance of the start time, so that the anxiety of being late does not add to the anxiety of presenting. Some conferences provide speaker rooms to enable a final check of AV aids and even a rehearsal of the talk.

During the presentation the presenter should remember to make eye contact with the audience, smile, and talk to the audience not the screen. They should check the audience's reactions and respond accordingly, for example giving further explanation if the audience does not seem to understand a point. Finally, the presenter should remember to speak clearly and slowly.

Dealing with anxiety

It is normal to feel anxious about a presentation. Anxiety is potentially useful as it will increase arousal, but too much anxiety can cripple. Extra chemical arousal from coffee, for example, is probably not going to be helpful. To minimize anxiety and its negative effects a presenter needs to accept that presentations are stressful, learn and use relaxation techniques, and use positive self-talk and visualization. It is useful to remember that the presenter will usually know what they did in their study better than anyone else, and that most audiences will assume that the research was good. Thus, if the AV aids are good, the content is well prepared and the presentation has been practised sufficiently, the presenter should be confident of success.

Question time

Novice presenters sometimes concentrate on the paper presentation to such an extent that on the day of delivery they present the paper well but lose control and reputation by not dealing well with question time. A good presenter prepares for questions as thoroughly as for the presentation. They should try to anticipate questions and get colleagues to anticipate questions, to which answers should be prepared. If there is some doubt whether questions will be asked, it is wise to arrange for some of the audience to have useful questions to initiate discussion.

A useful start to answering a question is to repeat a condensed version of it, especially if some of the audience might not have heard (sometimes the chairperson may repeat the question; see Chapter 22, p. 188). Responses should be brief, as most discussion times are very limited and the presenter will usually learn some useful feedback from questions. The presenter should answer the question and not use the opportunity as an excuse to deliver part two of the paper.

Most questions will be genuine queries to which a presenter will have a useful concise answer. However, if the answer is not known the presenter should not be afraid to say that they do not have an answer, and an offer should be extended to meet with the questioner to discuss the issue. Similarly, if an answer cannot be given succinctly and will be of little interest to the majority of the audience, the presenter should again offer to meet the questioner to discuss the details. If a question is not understood, the presenter should either ask for it to be repeated or suggest a meeting with the questioner after the session. Where a short answer is possible this is preferable to enable further valuable questions to be asked.

Unfortunately, some questioners will not be asking valid queries in a dispassionate way, which is the accepted scientific manner. If a member of the audience uses question time to self-promote, but does not really ask a question, the presenter can either ignore the comment and go on to the next person or say *Sorry, what was the question?* A good chairperson will usually deal with these people. Similarly, if a questioner is hostile a presenter should not respond in kind but rather remind the audience (and the hostile person in particular) that scientific knowledge is being discussed, which is always tentative. A similar response can be used if a questioner disagrees with the presenter, or makes a comment with which the presenter disagrees.

Hazard 19.3

Trying to present an inadequately prepared presentation

Failing to thoroughly check AV and prompt notes prior to leaving for presentation

Failing to prepare for equipment malfunction

This chapter has provided details to help the researching therapist prepare for and deliver a presentation which will meet the needs of the situation and enhance their professional reputation.

Further Reading

Calnan B 1972 Speaking at medical meetings. Heinemann, London

Eamon, M, Radloff A Teaching Learning Group, Curtin University, Personal Communication

Leeds, D 1988 Powerspeak: the complete guide to public speaking and presentations. Piaktus, London

Mandel S 1987 Effective presentation skills. Crisp Publications, Los Altos, California

Morris L L, Fitz-Gibbon C T, Freeman M E 1987 How to communicate evaluation findings. Sage Publications, Thousand Oaks

Murphy E 1992 Fear of lecturing: how to fly through. Campus Review 2(5), Feb 13–19

Newble D 1989 Making a presentation at a conference. In: A handbook for teachers in universities and colleges. Kogan Page, London

Presentation skills. Speak for yourself. BBC Training Videos

Richards I 1988 How to give a successful presentation: a concise guide for every manager. Graham and Trotman, London

Windschuttle K, Elliot E 1994 Writing, researching, communicating: communication skills for the information age, 2nd edn. McGraw-Hill, Sydney

20 Attending a scientific conference

Scientific conferences are an important mechanism for keeping up to date with recent developments, establishing contacts with key colleagues and for developing a profile and a reputation.

Besides presenting a paper at a conference, as discussed in Chapter 19, there are several other important professional skills associated with conference attendance. This chapter provides practical advice on how to set goals for conference attendance, how to choose a suitable conference to attend and how to prepare to make the maximum use of attendance. It also describes how conferences are typically organized and what changes are likely to occur in the next few years in how conferences are conducted. Chapter 21 describes how to prepare a poster for a conference and Chapter 22 discusses how to chair a session at a conference.

GOALS OF CONFERENCE ATTENDANCE

It is useful for researchers to identify their goals when planning to attend a conference. Common goals for new researchers would include obtaining information about the current state of knowledge; gaining impressions of the competence of colleagues; beginning to develop a network of colleagues with whom to collaborate; exposing their research to peer review; and developing a profile and a reputation.

Conferences provide an excellent opportunity to acquire information about the current state of knowledge in a particular area. Journal manuscripts are commonly submitted several years prior to publishing and are based on research conducted several years before that. Thus, articles published in 2002 may report on research conducted in 1998. Conferences have a much shorter lead time, enabling the findings of research conducted in the previous 2 years to be communicated.

This is important for a number of reasons. For example, attending a conference while in the initial stages of choosing or developing a research question can be a very valuable way of finding out about contemporary research. Similarly, important research findings can also affect clinical practice more rapidly via conferences.

However, the more rapid communication possible via conferences comes with costs. These include a more limited audience and a less detailed paper. Thus, sufficient detail may not be available to allow adequate peer review, and peer review may not be as stringent.

Conferences also provide an excellent opportunity to meet, and further assess the competence of, the authors of important papers. In discussions with such people it is usually possible to discern the level of understanding the person has both of the topic and of the limitations of their research. It is also possible to gain an impression of the author's attitude to scientific rigour. For example, a paper may read very well and appear to be describing very good research, and the reader may give some weight to the conclusions outlined in the paper. However, if when discussing this research with the author it is apparent that they have a limited understanding of the literature, a poor appreciation of the limitations of their methods and a less than rigorous attitude to research, the reader is likely to be less convinced by the conclusions in the written paper.

Having a network of colleagues who can be respected for their knowledge and understanding is an extremely useful resource for any researcher. By meeting and discussing research with colleagues at conferences a network of contacts can be developed.

Preliminary results are rarely publishable in journals. However, many conferences encourage the presentation of preliminary data. Researchers therefore use conference presentations to gain valuable peer review of theoretical concepts, methods and research findings.

Developing a profile and reputation via journal articles is important for a new researcher. A very good reputation can be developed by publication in quality journals, but this is usually a very lengthy process. Thus, presenting papers or posters and participating in discussions at conferences is an important and very quick way of developing a professional profile.

Conference attendance is costly in terms of time and money, so it needs to be effective. By choosing and participating in the right conference, optimal use of the time and money invested can be achieved.

CHOOSING A CONFERENCE

Each year new conferences appear and the choice of which conference to attend can be bewildering. Choosing the wrong conference will mean a waste of financial and time resources, whereas choosing the right one provides the opportunity for considerable learning and professional development.

The first step is to develop a list of potentially suitable conferences. Professional journals and newsletters usually contain notices of forthcoming conferences. Local professional and educational libraries can be used to search for the proceedings of relevant conferences by using subject and keyword indexes. The recommendations of colleagues are another good source. An increasing number of conferences are now advertised on the Internet. Often pages on the World Wide Web (WWW) are dedicated to information about a specific conference and others list conferences on various topics. Conferences are also advertised on the Internet via electronic discussion groups (e.g. Biomech-l, ErgonOz, Physio). To access this information it is necessary to subscribe to groups of related interest and either wait for information or ask the group for ideas.

The second step in choosing a conference is to assess each one. Two aspects of a conference should be assessed before deciding which to attend: the quality and relevance of the papers and discussion, and the time, place and cost.

Quality and relevance of a conference

To evaluate the quality and relevance of papers at a conference past proceedings should be reviewed. The amount of detail provided (often very restricted at a conference) should be considered, as should the quality of the research presented. Sometimes it is possible to assess the quality of the work presented at a conference by seeing if some of the papers are subsequently published in quality journals. It may also be possible to establish who attends a conference. By viewing who presented, and if possible who attended (attendance lists may be available from colleagues who have previously attended the conference), it is possible to see if the relevant leading researchers and clinicians attend. This helps provide an indication of the level of discussion one can expect.

Time, place and cost of a conference

Invariably there are constraints over when one may be able to attend a conference. The location should also be considered, as this will affect travelling time and also travel and accommodation costs. (For many the lure of an exotic location may be the deciding factor.) The registration costs for conferences vary greatly and may preclude some conferences.

Hazard 20.1

Selecting a conference without adequate background information

EFFECTIVE USE OF CONFERENCE ATTENDANCE

Once a suitable conference has been chosen, several important aspects should be considered to ensure effective use of attendance. These include presenting, selecting suitable sessions, participating in formal and informal discussions and identifying key colleagues.

As previously stated, optimum gain at conferences comes not only from hearing presentations but from participation. This includes presenting a verbal paper or poster, asking questions and making comments during formal discussions following paper presentations, asking questions and making comments during formal discussions at poster presentations and informal discussions with colleagues.

Presenting a paper well is an excellent way to demonstrate one's competence: other attendees will be more willing to spend their valuable time in discussions with someone who has demonstrated competence in the area (see Chapter 19 for advice on presentation of a paper and Chapter 21 for advice on preparing a poster).

Many conferences run multiple sessions concurrently and the sessions should be carefully chosen to obtain maximum value. Some conferences publish a programme and distribute it well ahead of the date, whereas programmes for other conferences are only available upon registration. Either way, an opportunity exists to review the programme and select which sessions to attend. Most sessions chosen are likely to be in one's main area of interest; however, allowance should be made for some attendance at sessions peripheral to one's usual specialty area. Listening to several papers is an easy way to find out what is happening in other areas. Often serendipitous attendance at an unrelated session will provide new insights, models and methods which can be applied to one's own main area of interest.

Participating in formal discussions, when there is an audience listening to what is said, is also an excellent opportunity to demonstrate understanding and competence. Care should be taken to not appear boastful, grandiose or hypercritical, as this will alienate colleagues. Formal discussion time is usually very short, so questions should be concise. If an issue will take considerable time to discuss adequately, it is recommended to suggest to the presenter that those interested can meet after the session.

The informal discussions over breaks, meals and social activities are often the most valuable part of a conference – something one cannot get from the published proceedings. Opportunities for such informal discussions can be planned for by identifying suitable times and key people. Some conferences provide a list of attendees upon registration, and a good practice is to review this list and highlight the key colleagues to speak with. During the conference the list can be referred to regularly to ensure that desired contacts are made. Also, upon registering, the programme should be reviewed to identify suitable times for informal discussions.

If possible, contact with key colleagues should be made prior to the conference to establish a relationship and plan the exchange of papers or ideas. This will help make optimal use of the short time available for face-to-face discussions.

CONFERENCE ORGANIZATION

Scientific conferences can be confusing for the new participant. However, as most follow a similar pattern, a brief review of typical conference organization will help new participants understand the process.

Conferences are typically advertised for 1–3 years beforehand; major international conferences have longer notification times to allow people to start preparing funding and free time early. Most quality conferences will call for abstracts of papers to be submitted up to 6–12 months prior to the start date. Abstracts then undergo peer review and authors are informed whether their paper has been accepted, and if so whether it is to be presented verbally or as a poster (sometimes the author is given the choice). Verbal papers are generally considered more prestigious than poster papers, although the latter can often generate better discussion.

Successful authors are sent specifications for the presentation of their paper and its publication. Thus the authors of a verbal paper should be informed how long the presentations are, how long question time will be, who will chair their session, and the types of audiovisual equipment available. Authors of posters should be informed of the required size and the mechanism for display. Conferences usually publish either the abstracts or full written papers as the proceedings, and authors should be notified of the detailed requirements for these.

The standards of conference organization are quite variable, partly because most conferences move to a new geographical location each time. The organizing committees are thus often arranging the conference for the first time. A well-organized conference will enable the researcher to gain the maximum benefit from attendance. Apart from understanding how conferences are currently organized, it will be useful for the researching therapist to have an awareness of how conferences may change in the near future.

THE FUTURE OF CONFERENCES

Fora for the exchange of scientific information are becoming increasingly important owing to the increasing depth of knowledge expected (due to the expanding knowledge base available) and the increasing breadth of knowledge expected (due to the increasing complexity of research designs and the trend for multidisciplinary investigation of research problems). The necessity for therapists to be up to date in this expanding sea of knowledge is likely to increase the importance of conferences in the foreseeable future.

The need to exchange scientific information rapidly has resulted in an escalation in the number of conferences likely to be of interest to therapists. This, together with inevitable financial considerations, will continue to make careful selection of, and preparation for, conferences important. The rapid developments in information technology provide additional mechanisms for information exchange, and hence new opportunities for researching therapists wishing to keep up to date.

More information becomes available to the researching therapist daily via the Internet. Electronic mail is becoming more pervasive and offers excellent opportunities for geographically separated colleagues to discuss issues without exorbitant costs. Collaboration is now made easy with data, document and comment communication via the Internet. Electronic discussion groups (e.g. Biomech-l, ErgoNet, PTeduc) also provide new opportunities for therapists to participate in scientific discussions. Besides providing an alternative to physical conference attendance, these developments in information technology also enable attendees to be better informed prior to arriving at a conference, and thus better able to use conference time effectively.

One recent development set to radically change the way scientific conferences are used is the virtual conference. A virtual conference takes place in cyberspace, that is, rather than being located in a specific geographical location, it is conducted over the Internet. Papers are 'presented' as text, graphics, sound and video. People 'attend' the conference by connecting to it via their desktop computers. Conference 'attendees'

then interact with the presenter and each other, asking questions, providing answers and adding comments, just as one would at a 'flesh' conference. Figure 20.1 shows the computer screen for a recent virtual conference, CybErg 1996 (CybErg can be viewed on the WWW at: http://www.curtin.edu.au/conference/cyberg).

Two aspects of virtual conferences are especially noteworthy: cost and discussion time.

As there is no physical travel involved in attending virtual conferences, the expense associated with travel fares and accommodation is avoided, and as there are no venues to hire the conference running costs, and hence the registration costs, can also be significantly lower. All that

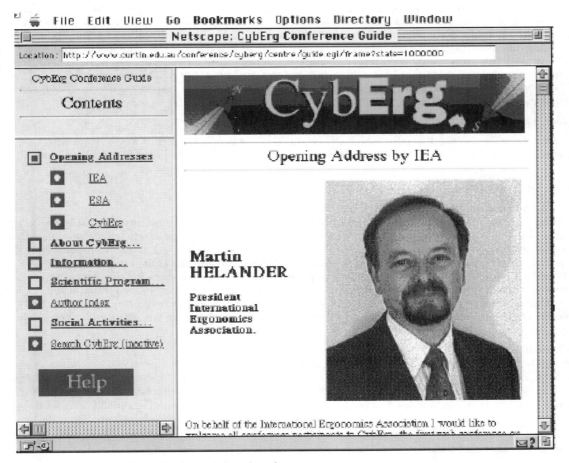

Figure 20.1 A view of the CybErg 1996 virtual conference

Discussion Topic

How can VDT users use the research results on mice?
Hongzheng Lu (Sat, 14 Sep 1996 03:22:24 GMT)

Assume that you found a significant increase in muscle load in certain muscle groups after investigating a large subject sample. The results indicated that the risk of wrist/shoulder/arm injuries increased when using a mouse. So what? Are you going to recommend VDT users not use the mice? For a lot of tasks, mice can significantly improve work efficiency. Just some thoughts.
- Cindy

List of Responses

Systematic approach to risk control
Leon Straker (Mon, 16 Sep 1996 01:19:57 GMT)

Thanks for query Cindy,
Our approach to risk control is to first identify the hazard (what this pilot study and its follow up will do to see if there is a problem). If early indications are that it is likely to contribute to the risk of work related musculoskeletal disorders we would look in more detail - Risk Assessment, and trial some interventions to control identified contributors to risk - Risk Control. Currently software design, in my opinion, is technology and market driven - mice exist, the consumers buy programmes mouse driven so programmers produce mouse oriented programmes. Currently this takes no account for potential MSD problems. To answer your 'So, what?' - if mouse use is shown to increase the risk of MSD, then some of the following could be useful:
* trialing different furniture design to better accommodate mouse use (see Hamilton paper); * guidelines to software designers on location of features on screen to reduce difficult movements/excessive mouse kilometerage (see current trend to put clickable controls on tool bars at top AND bottom of screen;
* guidelines to users on risks and suggestions of appropriate work practices etc. Hopefully that has given you some idea on how the results of this study could be practically used.

Hongzheng Lu (Mon, 16 Sep 1996 04:24:27 GMT)

Thanks, Leon. I also think that education is important. Training people the correct way to work with computers to reduce physical and mental stress is as important as giving the user a better design mouse.

The cost of mousing
Annabel Cooper (Wed, 18 Sep 1996 10:19:11 GMT)

Thanks for another interesting topic of discussion, Cindy.
Although mousing may increase efficiency for some tasks, if the cost of that efficiency eventually results in significant injuries, perhaps the cost of efficiency is rather high? Some suggestions to reduce possible excessive muscular load during mouse use may include: ensuring that the workstation is properly set up for the individual user in order to maintain a neutral shoulder position with the entire forearm supported; alternating sides for mousing so that the load is spread between both sides; ensuring that the user takes regular breaks from the repetitive activity of mousing; replacing mousing with learned bilateral key commands whenever appropriate; and perhaps eventually using voice-activated computer systems that require neither excessive use of the mouse or the keyboard - wouldn't that be nice! Does anyone else have any further suggestions or comments?

Alternative devices
Robin Burgess-Limerick (Fri, 20 Sep 1996 01:34:20 GMT)
What about alternative pointing devices. I find the mouse gives me a pain in the wrist from too much ulnar deviation, so I alternate between touch pad, graphics tablet, and two different track balls. None is perfect, and each takes a bit of getting used to, but the variation seems to avoid the pain! I'm still looking for the perfect device, but it may be, like seated posture, that there is no such animal and that variation is the key.

Figure 20.2 Sample of discussion from CybErg 1996

is required is a desktop computer and access to the Internet. These can be acquired in most places for less than the cost of attendance at one international conference.

One of the most dissatisfying aspects of 'flesh' conferences is the pressure of time. This makes paper presentations short and discussions brief. Virtual conferences can run for several weeks, allowing adequate time for authors to consider questions fully and even provide further data and analysis. This provides a much better quality and depth of discussion than is possible with the usual time constraints at conferences. (Some conferences are also trying to improve the quality of the discussion by restricting presentation time and allowing more time for discussion.) Figure 20.2 shows some discussion from the first virtual conference on the WWW, CybErg 1996.

Further Reading

Maitland I 1996 How to organise a conference. Gower, Aldershot

Key Points 20.1

Know one's goals before selecting a conference

Prepare for maximum use of conference time

Refer back to aims of attendance during conference

Use new technologies to supplement traditional conferences

These two aspects of virtual conferences thus allow the researching therapist to attend a greater number of better, international-quality conferences. Naturally, virtual interaction is not as satisfying as face-to-face communication, but it provides a powerful adjunct to the opportunities available to the researching therapist.

This chapter suggested how to select a conference and gain maximum benefit from attendance. It also provided an overview of how conferences are typically organised and gave a glimpse of what the future of conferences may look like. The following two chapters present details of other aspects of conference participation.

21

Preparing a conference poster

CHAPTER CONTENTS

Posters convey a strong visual message and are one of the simplest and most direct forms of communication. A research poster should be designed to attract the reader's attention, giving them a desire to investigate further. The factors that contribute to a successful poster include: the art of concise writing; thoughtful organization, effective layout design and use of visual material; an understanding of the message that is to be conveyed; and knowledge of the audience that will view the poster.

A poster has a different function from that of a verbal conference presentation. Whereas the verbal presentation generally has a wider audience and some opportunity for questions, time constraints often do not allow in-depth discussion of the methods or results. In contrast, posters are more likely to attract interested parties who wish to discuss the research in more depth with the presenter. Many conferences include a formal poster session where presenters are expected to be available for discussion. If a formal session is not organized the presenter should make themselves available during key viewing times, such as breaks between sessions.

This chapter outlines the information that should be included on a poster, and discusses how to design and construct a poster.

CONTENT

As posters are a visual medium the author should aim to present the information in a manner which is likely to attract and maintain the interest of the audience. Elements which attract attention are areas of large text such as the title, and graphics such as photographs, diagrams and graphs. To keep the reader's attention, large sections of text should be avoided and diagrams and graphs kept as simple as possible.

In each of the sections of the poster only the main points should be presented. Economy of words is required, as there is limited space available. Important points such as the aims or purpose of the study can be emphasized using bulleted lists (generally preceded by a symbol such as •), which draw attention and are easier to read than complete sentences or large blocks of text.

The poster is generally divided into seven main sections: title, byline, introduction, methods, results, conclusions and acknowledgements. These sections are described in more detail below. Some variation in the number and content of these sections may be required, depending on the type of research being reported, the type of conference and the background of the intended audience.

Title

The title for a poster differs from the type of title used for a paper. It should be short (no more than 12 words) and phrased to capture the reader's interest. Owing to the large font size needed to make it stand out, the title may span one or two widths of the poster. If two lines are required the words should be grouped to create an even balance between the line lengths. When typesetting the title the first letter of each word should be capitalized (excluding small words such as 'the', 'and', 'of'). Alternatively, the whole title may be capitalized; however, this may increase the line length and will make the title more difficult to read, particularly from a distance (see Appendix E).

Byline

The byline contains the authors' names and is placed below the title. It may also include each author's title (Dr, Professor), designation (stu-

dent, supervisor) and institutional affiliation. Posters presented by students should include two bylines: the first should contain the name of the student and the second the name of the supervisor, each with the appropriate designations.

Introduction

This section should be brief, aiming to provide the reader with the main points required to understand the statement of the problem. This then leads to a presentation of the purpose (or aims) of the study.

Methods

In providing a description of the methods the following components should be covered, but in much less detail than is required for a written paper: study design; description of subjects, variables (including operational definitions of dependent, independent and extraneous variables); and testing procedures (see Chapters 5 and 18 for further details).

Results

Results that are presented in graphic or tabular form are easier than blocks of text for the reader to take in quickly, and also make the poster more attractive. When reporting the results of statistical analyses the type of statistical procedure which was performed should be clearly identified. For example, $F_{(1,13)}=2.4$; $P = 0.02$ makes it clear that an analysis of variance was used with two groups and 14 subjects.

Conclusions

The aims of the study and the conclusions are the two main focus points on a poster. If these two components are presented in a clear and concise fashion the reader will be able to quickly ascertain whether the research is of interest to them. This may then lead to further discussion with the authors. As with the introduction, the conclusions may be presented in point form.

Acknowledgements

The acknowledgement section may be printed in a smaller type size as it is not critical to the understanding of the research. The following information may be included: a statement which indicates that the research received ethical approval; a statement that indicates whether the research was performed as part of the requirement for a course or degree; acknowledgements of financial assistance from grants or scholarships; the names of individuals who provided key assistance during the research but are not included in the byline; and the date of the conference or poster presentation.

DESIGN

When designing the layout of the poster there are two factors to consider. The first and most important relates to the size and dimensions of the poster. These are generally as recommended by the conference organizers. Occasionally, the space allocated to each poster will be given, rather than the recommended dimensions. If the space extends from the floor, the bottom 0.75 m should not be used as the reader will not be able to see this area easily while standing.

The second factor to consider is the layout of the poster presentation area, as this will determine the viewing distance (distance between poster and reader). Such information is seldom provided to the authors but the following guidelines will suit most situations. Although the main text is generally read from a distance of 1–2 m, the headings and title should be large enough to be viewed from further away. The recommended type sizes for the various text components are shown in Table 21.1.

Once the dimensions of the poster have been determined a design layout can be planned. The following discussion uses the design principle of a grid. The grid system utilizes a series of vertical and horizontal lines that divide the layout into parts and act as guides for the placement of text and graphics. The grid provides the underlying structure for the poster. Using the grid system the same poster can be designed to fit on a single

Table 21.1 Recommended font sizes for poster presentations

	Viewing distance (m)	Type size (pt)*
Title	5	60–108
Byline	3	36–48
Headings	3	36–54
Text	1–2	18–24
Acknowledgements	1	12–14

* 1 pt ~ 0.35 mm

large 'page', or be broken up into smaller pieces for easier transport to the venue.

As in a journal or newspaper, the information on a poster is generally organized into columns. However, unlike the information printed on a standard page, which is viewed close up, the information on a poster is also viewed from a distance. Consequently there are two lines of sight, or paths the reader follows through the information presented (Fig. 21.1). From a distance the eye will tend to scan from the top left corner to the bottom right corner, but when close up will follow the normal reading pattern, moving from the top of the column to the bottom and from the left column to the right (this pattern may differ between cultures). The grid used for a poster should take advantage of these scanning patterns to direct the reader's attention from the aims of the project (placed in the top left corner) to the conclusions (placed in the bottom right corner). Any graphics or elements of interest should also be placed on this line. The basic components of a grid system for designing a poster are detailed in Figure 21.1.

The actual dimensions of the poster to some extent determine the layout grid that can be used. A poster that is presented in landscape format, which is wider than it is tall, can accommodate more columns than one presented in portrait format, which is taller than it is wide. The following discussion will consider a poster measuring 102 cm wide by 81 cm high.

The two most functional layout grids are the three-column grid (Fig. 21.2) and the four-column grid (Fig. 21.3). The three-column grid

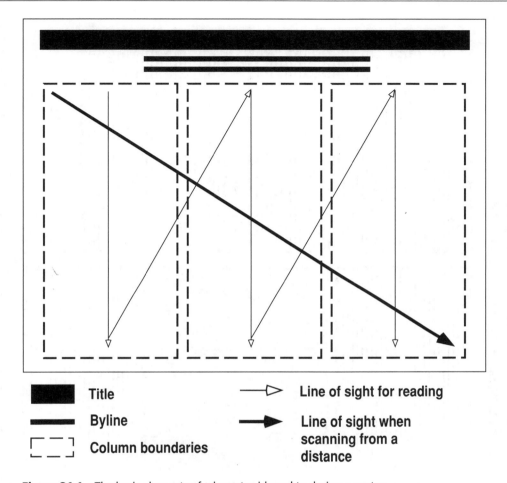

Figure 21.1   The basic elements of a layout grid used to design a poster

incorporates a single graphic element placed along the scanning line in the centre of the poster. This grid is suitable for posters which require large amounts of text. Blocks of text can be printed on standard A4 paper in landscape format which corresponds to the column width. If two or more graphics are to be included a four-column grid should be used. The graphics are then placed diagonally on the scanning line, or are grouped in the centre. Text can be printed on A4 paper in portrait format.

CONSTRUCTION

Colour is an important tool that can be used effectively to attract attention to the poster and to add style; colour can also be misused (see discussion on the use of colour in Chapter 19, p. 166). The most obvious colour element on a poster is the background, but graphics can also be presented in colour. If colour graphics are used the background should be subtle (grey or neutral), complementing the primary colour elements of the graphic. Colours which clash or are too close in tone to the graphic material should be avoided. If the graphics are black and white or grey scale, a bolder background colour can be used. In either situation only a single colour should be used for the background, as multiple colours will tend to divide rather than unite the elements of

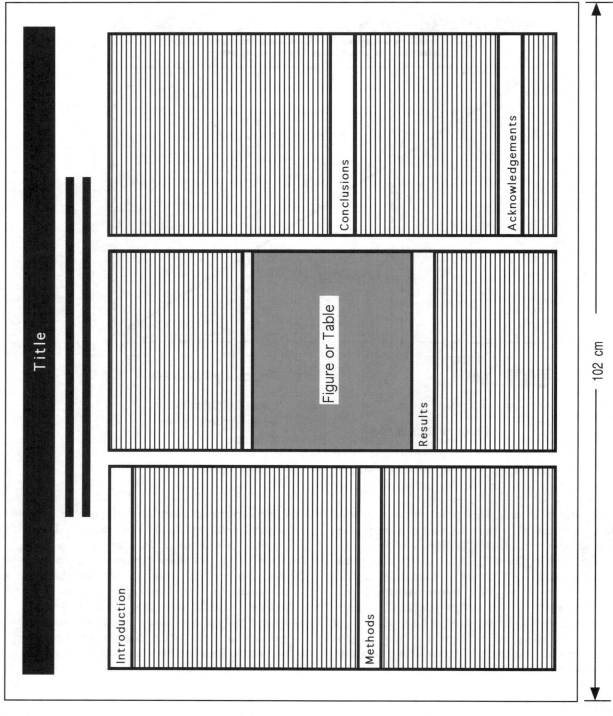

Figure 21.2   Layout for a poster using a three-column grid

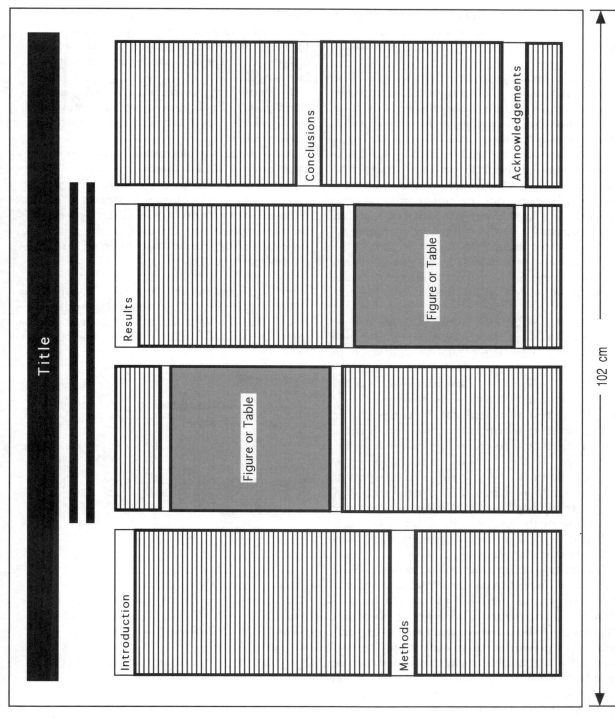

Figure 21.3   Layout for a poster using a four-column grid

the poster. Thin boundary strips can be used around graphic elements, or around the poster to provide contrast and to give it a more professional look.

The title, headings and text blocks should be printed in black on white or light-coloured paper. Sans serif fonts are best as they have a clean crisp appearance and are easy to read from a distance (see Appendix E for examples).

Unless the poster must be rolled up the background material should be stiff (1–2 mm thick) to hold its shape when mounted and to prevent creasing. Most posters are constructed on card or mounting board, but any suitable material can be used. To mount the paper on the background spray mounting adhesive should be used, as this provides a good even contact without warping the paper. It also allows the paper to be peeled off and repositioned if necessary.

As desktop publishing software becomes more widely available an increasing number of posters will be generated using this technology. These programs allow the poster to be laid out on a single 'page' of the correct dimensions, and special layout commands provide increased flexibility for placing text and graphics. The computer file is then taken to a printer for colour production. This method may be costly: the cost will generally depend on the size of the page and the number of colours to be printed. Photographs or other graphics must be either created in a digital format or digitized using an image scanner. The resolution of the image is important as images with low resolutions may look grainy, particularly if they are enlarged.

The method of construction will depend on the mode of transport to the presentation venue. If the conference is local the poster can be constructed in one piece on large poster boards. If the poster is to be presented at a national or international conference it will be easier to transport if mounted on a flexible background that can be rolled and stored in a poster tube, or mounted on smaller segments of poster board which can later be placed beside each other like pieces of a puzzle. If a modular approach is used the segments should be of the same size, except for the title,

which can be constructed in one piece to maintain good alignment. For transport the mounting board behind the title section can be cut with a scalpel, leaving the plastic laminate intact to act as a hinge.

To ensure that the poster arrives at its destination intact the final product should be laminated; a matt finish is preferable, to reduce glare from overhead lighting.

If the poster is to be mounted on a smooth surface double-sided adhesive which is easily removed should be used in preference to pins or tacks, which will leave permanent marks. Adhesive Velcro strips are ideal: if the hook component is placed on the back of the mounting board the poster can be easily hung on cloth-covered display panels.

A well designed poster that is visually appealing will attract interested viewers and stimulate further discussion with the author(s), thus achieving the aim of communicating the research findings.

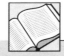 **Further Reading**

Briscoe M H 1990 A researcher's guide to scientific and medical illustrations. Springer-Verlag, New York

Harms M 1995 How to ... prepare a poster presentation. Physiotherapy 81(5): 276–277

Shushan R ,Wright D, Birmele R 1991 Desktop publishing by design. Microsoft Press, Redmond, Washington

22 Chairing a session at a conference

This chapter discusses the important role of the chairperson and provides guidelines to assist in chairing a session at a conference.

The success of a free paper session (i.e. one that comprises a series of presentations, often on related topics and given by different presenters) or one consisting of presentations from invited speakers depends not only on the quality of the presentations but also to a large extent on how well the session is conducted by the chairperson. Being present at a session in which the chairperson allows speakers to exceed their allotted time is a frustrating experience, as is the failure of the chairperson to conduct the discussion in an efficient and orderly manner. Where a conference consists of several concurrent sessions and the scheduled times for the presentations are not strictly adhered to, members of the audience may miss out on hearing presentations in other sessions. Thorough preparation by the chairperson is essential to the smooth running and success of a session.

RESPONSIBILITIES OF THE CHAIRPERSON

The chairperson has responsibilities to the organizers of the conference, the speakers and the audience (Newble & Cannon 1989).

Responsibilities to the organizers

It is the chairperson's responsibility to ensure that any instructions or requests from the organizers are carried out. The organizers should provide the chairperson with a programme for the session, identify whether there are concurrent sessions and send a copy of any instructions given to the speakers. If this information is not forthcoming it is the responsibility of the chairperson to seek it out. Instructions for the conduct of the session may also be provided. The chairperson may also receive the contact details and curricula vitae of the speakers; this generally occurs when a session has one or more invited speakers. The organizers may ask the chairperson to contact the speakers in the weeks prior to the conference to outline the conduct of the session. For international conferences contact is usually made immediately prior to the meeting. At this time it may also be relevant to discuss the points the chairperson intends to make when introducing the speaker(s).

Responsibilities to the speakers

Responsibilities include familiarizing the speakers with the required audiovisual equipment and the method to be used to time the session, and to notify the speaker of the time remaining. During the discussion period the chairperson must ensure fair play: this may include suggesting that lengthy discussions of major differences of opinion are reserved for breaks between sessions. The chairperson is responsible for ensuring that questioners do not make mini presentations of their own research.

Responsibilities to the audience

The main responsibilities of the chairperson to the audience are to ensure that they can hear the speaker and see any visual presentations; to keep the speakers on time, thereby preserving time for questions; to ensure that question time is not dominated by one member of the audience; and to initiate discussion by asking a question if none are forthcoming.

Occasionally two chairpersons may be appointed, in which case it is necessary to decide how the role of each is to be defined: for example, one may open and the other close the session.

The chairpersons may be responsible for introducing alternate speakers and for moderating the ensuing discussions.

The following guidelines are designed to assist the chairperson of a free paper session and sessions consisting of one or more invited speakers. The first series of guidelines outline the procedures which need to be taken prior to the session. This is followed by a section addressing the conduct of the session. The last two sections provide guidelines for chairing the discussion and for concluding the session. Suggested phraseology is given in italics.

PRIOR TO THE SESSION

The chairperson needs to carefully read the programme for the session and, where available, the abstracts of the presentations or the summary provided by a keynote speaker (a keynote speaker is usually a leading authority in a particular area of research or clinical practice). It may be useful to prepare a few questions or comments for each abstract or summary. If answers are not provided during the presentation these may comprise the standby questions to be used to initiate the discussion when necessary.

It is essential that the chairperson is familiar with the venue. If time allows, this may include observing an earlier session conducted in the same venue, or a survey of the venue prior to the first session on the day. When this is not possible, the chairperson needs to arrive at the session room at least 15 minutes before the scheduled starting time. When surveying the venue the chairperson should pay attention to the following:

- Note the placement of the lectern for the speaker.
- Note the place allocated for the chairperson to sit, ensuring that this allows a clear view of the speaker and audiovisual presentations.
- Check the visual angles from several points within the venue to identify any areas where the audience should be advised not to sit.
- Ensure that there is water available both for the speakers and for the chairperson.

- Become familiar with the operation of the equipment supplied to the speaker, such as the pointer, microphone, the remote control for slides and the controls for any other audiovisual equipment (e.g. overhead projector, video player, computer projection system).
- Note the timing mechanism to be used to inform speakers of the time remaining and when they must finish.

The extent to which the chairperson needs to be familiar with the audiovisual equipment and the controls for the lighting (e.g. to enable dimming of the lights during the presentation) will vary depending on the level of technical support provided. The chairperson may be responsible for demonstrating to the speakers the operation of the audiovisual equipment. At many conferences, technical staff or members of the organizing committee are assigned to control the lighting and to deal with any malfunctioning of equipment. However, it is strongly recommended that the chairperson check the operation of the equipment and become familiar with the controls, at least for the equipment used by the speakers (e.g. slide projector or overhead projector). After doing this, the chairperson should seek out and introduce him/herself to the speakers and confirm the type of audiovisual equipment each will be using. For presentations using 35 mm slides, the chairperson must ensure that each speaker has loaded their slides in a carousel and given the carousel to the projectionist, if one is present. The chairperson should then ask the speakers to sit at the front of the room, as this minimizes time lost during the changeover between papers.

Different methods are used at conferences to signal the end of the presentation time. Among the more sophisticated is a series of lights on the lectern to inform speakers of the amount of time remaining. Other methods include a buzzer or bell, which is sounded when only 1–2 minutes remain and repeated at the end of the time. Alternatively, the chairperson may raise a card showing the number of minutes remaining. The chairperson should assume the responsibility for clearly explaining to the speakers the method which will be used.

THE SESSION

The session must start promptly at the specified time. Each presentation must also commence at the listed time: a delay, however short, will cause problems. In the event that a speaker fails to appear, the chairperson should apologize to the audience and then wait until the scheduled time for the next paper. To do otherwise is unfair to delegates who may be intending to hear only part of the scheduled session. If concurrent sessions are not programmed, it may be acceptable to continue with the next presentation and not wait until the scheduled time. The potential problem of what to do if a speaker fails to appear should be outlined in advance by the conference organizers; failing this, it is wise for the chairperson to seek clarification on this issue.

A total of 15–20 minutes is the usual time allowed for an oral presentation. This may comprise 10–15 minutes for the speaker to deliver the paper, 4 minutes for the discussion, and 1 minute for the changeover and introduction. Alternatively, a 20-minute period may be divided equally between the presentation and the discussion. In some sessions a number of papers are presented and discussion is reserved until all presentations have been given. The time allowed for a presentation from a keynote speaker varies, but is commonly in the order of 40–60 minutes, followed by a 10–20 minute period for discussion.

The introduction

Before introducing the first speaker, the chairperson is responsible for officially opening the session and extending a welcome to the audience. The introduction should state the topic of the session and the guidelines for the discussion time. For example:

I would like to welcome you to this session on the management of motor learning difficulties in children. This session will consist of three 15-minute papers. Following each paper there will be 4 minutes for ques-

tions on that paper. Please reserve your questions on each paper until the respective question time. When you wish to ask a question, please move towards a floor microphone, identify yourself by name, institution, city and country, and speak slowly and clearly into the microphone.

If neither a floor microphone nor a roving microphone is available, the chairperson should request that those with a question stand and speak loudly, slowly and clearly.

For speakers of free papers, 1 minute is generally allowed for the introduction and changeover. As the speaker approaches the lectern, the chairperson introduces the speaker, reads the title of the paper, the names of any co-authors and the name of the institution(s). For example:

The next paper is by Smith, Frank and White from the School of Occupational Therapy, the Western University, Perth, Western Australia. The title of the paper is `An analysis of the employment trends of occupational therapists'. Sonia Smith will present the paper.

For keynote speakers it is reasonable to provide a longer introduction, usually in the order of 2–3 minutes. This should include the name and position of the speaker and other information as appropriate, for example details of their area of expertise and key publications. To assist with this, keynote speakers are usually asked to provide a short curriculum vitae which is made available to the chairperson well in advance of the session.

The discussion

At the end of each presentation the speaker should be thanked and the paper opened for discussion, for example: *Thank you Sonia Smith. This paper is now open for discussion.* At this point it may be necessary to remind those wishing to ask questions that they are required to stand, identify themselves and to speak clearly into a microphone (where available).

It may be necessary for the chairperson to start the discussion by asking one or two questions in the event that none are forthcoming from the audience. These will need to be formulated and written down during the presenta-

tion, or may have arisen earlier when reading the abstract.

Throughout the discussion the chairperson is required to ensure a fair order is used for taking the questions. The chairperson should try to take as many questions as is practical and ensure that one questioner does not dominate the entire discussion period. If an individual appears to have multiple questions it is reasonable to suggest that they speak with the presenter after the session. It is important to assess whether it might have been difficult for all the audience to hear the question, and if so the question should be repeated. At the end of the discussion, the chairperson should thank the speaker again and proceed to the next paper.

The conclusion

At the end of the session it is important to thank both the speakers and the members of the audience. For example:

This concludes the session on the management of low back pain. I would like to thank the speakers and the audience for their participation and attention.

Assuming the presentations have been interesting and of a high quality, then a comment to this effect should be included in the concluding remarks.

Sometimes the chairperson is asked to provide information of a more general nature before the audience leaves the venue. This may include information about a change in venue or starting time for a following session. Before leaving the venue, the speakers should be reminded to collect their slides from the projection room.

REFERENCE

Newble D, Cannon R 1989. A handbook for teachers in universities & colleges. Kogan Page, London

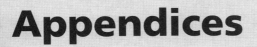

Appendices

Appendix A
Example: informed
consent documents

SUBJECT INFORMATION SHEET

Title of Project: The effects of arm exercises on breathing and heart rate in healthy males aged 40–60 years
Principal Investigator: I. M. Keen BSc (Physio.) Postgraduate student, School of Therapy, Western University. Tel 111-2000
Tel 111-2222 (after work hours)
Project Supervisor: Dr Academe PhD. Senior Lecturer, School of Therapy, Western University. Telephone 111-2000

Purpose of study
Patients undergoing surgery via a general anaesthetic are prone to developing lung complications in the first few days after operation. The gases breathed for the anaesthetic and the drugs given to relieve pain dry the normal lung fluids and inhibit the taking of deep breaths. When operations are performed on the abdomen, heart or lungs, patients are reluctant to cough or take deep breaths because of pain or fear of pain.

Physiotherapists have an important role in the prevention and treatment of these complications. Several different methods are used for this purpose, all of which aim to assist patients to take deep breaths and to remove any phlegm from the lungs. One of the simplest methods is encouraging patients to perform arm exercises, as these increase the depth of breathing and assist in the movement of oxygen around the body.

Although arm exercises are used by physiotherapists, researchers have not investigated the effects of the specific forms of exercises used by physiotherapists. Therefore, there is no information regarding the effects of such exercises on breathing or heart rate in healthy subjects or in postoperative patients.

You are invited to participate in a study which aims to determine the most effective form of arm exercise to be used with post-operative patients by investigating the effects of low-intensity arm exercise on breathing and heart rate in healthy subjects.

Procedures
If you are prepared to be involved in the study you will be required to attend the School of Therapy on two occasions not more than 1 week apart and at approximately the same time of the day. Prior to each visit it is essential that you do not eat any food for 2 hours or have any drinks which contain caffeine (tea or coffee) or alcohol. This is important as food and certain drinks can affect heart rate and breathing.

Visit 1
On the first visit your lung function will be measured by asking you to blow into a machine three times. This requires some effort but should not cause any discomfort. Also, your blood pressure will be recorded by placing an inflatable cuff around your arm. Heart rate will be measured using a cardiac monitor attached to the front of your chest by means of three small discs placed on the skin surface, occasionally it is necessary to shave a small amount of hair in order to achieve good contact. After these measurements have been made you will have a short trial run using the equipment that will be used to measure your breathing, and you will have an opportunity to practise the two types of arm exercises that will be investigated. Visit 1 will last no more than 1 hour.

Visit 2
All the measurements will be performed with you sitting in a chair with your feet resting on the floor. The heart rate monitor will be attached to your chest. The rate and depth of your breathing and the amount of oxygen and carbon dioxide you breathe out will be measured by asking you to breathe through a mouthpiece which is connected to a flow tube. As you must only breathe via your mouth, it is essential that you wear a nose clip.

After an initial rest period of 10 minutes, you will be asked to perform the first arm exercise for no longer than 4 minutes. This will be followed by another rest period of 5–10 minutes, after which time you will be asked to perform the second arm exercise, again for no more than four minutes. After the second exercise there will be another rest period of 5–10 minutes. Heart rate and breathing will be continuously measured throughout the rest and exercise periods. Visit 2 will last no more than 1 hour.

All measurements will be performed by the Principal Investigator and the studies will take place in the Exercise Science Laboratory at the School of Therapy.

Risks, discomforts and benefits
It is not anticipated that you will experience any discomfort from the exercises or any of the measurement procedures, except perhaps for very minimal discomfort for the first minute or so when breathing through the mouthpiece.

The exercises are designed for use with patients in the first few days after major operations and therefore are not physically demanding and so should not cause any undue tiredness. Testing will be terminated immediately upon your request, if you experience any undue discomfort or fatigue or if any abnormal responses to the exercises occur.

If you take part in this study you will learn about the place of upper limb exercises in the maintenance of fitness levels. The results we obtain in this study will be very important in helping to determine the most effective type of upper limb exercises for use in the physiotherapy management of postoperative patients.

Confidentiality
You will be allocated an identification number which will remain confidential to the Principal Investigator and the Project Supervisor. All the data recorded, using only the assigned number for identification, will be stored on a computer in the School of Therapy and access to the stored data will be restricted by a password known only to the Principal Investigator and the Project Supervisor. Data collection sheets and questionnaires will be stored in a locked cupboard.

The results of the study will be reported but it will not be possible to identify individual subjects. Once the study has been completed, the data will be stored with the Project Supervisor in a secure place for 5 years, after which time it will be destroyed. This is a requirement of Western University.

Request for more information
You are encouraged to discuss any concerns regarding the study with the Principal Investigator at any time, and to ask any questions you may have.

Refusal or withdrawal
You may refuse to participate in the study and if you do consent to participate then you will be free to withdraw from the study at any time and without fear of prejudice. If you do decide to withdraw from the study then please contact the Principal Investigator at the earliest opportunity. In the event that you withdraw, all your data will be destroyed.

CONSENT SHEET

Title of Project: The effects of arm exercises on breathing and heart rate in healthy males aged 40 to 60 years
Principal Investigator: I. M. Keen BSc (Physio.) Postgraduate student, School of Therapy, Western University.
                             Tel 111-2000; 111-2222 (after work hours)
Project Supervisor: Dr Academe PhD. Senior Lecturer, School of Therapy, Western University. Tel 111-2000

You are voluntarily making a decision whether or not to participate in this research study. Your signature certifies that you have decided to participate, having read and understood the information presented. Your signature also certifies that you have had an adequate opportunity to discuss this study with the investigator and you have had all your questions answered to your satisfaction. You will be given a copy of this consent form to keep.

I, (the undersigned) _____
                                                Please PRINT

of _____

Postcode _____   Phone _____

consent to participate in this study and give my permission for any results from this study to be used in any report or research paper, on the understanding that confidentiality will be preserved. I understand that I may withdraw from the study at any time without prejudice. If so, I undertake to contact the Principal Investigator (Tel. 351-3600) at the earliest opportunity.

Signature: _____   Date: _____
        Subject / Parent / Guardian / Custodian

I have explained the nature of and the procedures involved in the study to which the subject has consented to participate and have answered all questions. In my judgement the subject is voluntarily and knowingly giving informed consent and possesses the legal capacity to give informed consent to participate in this research study.

Principal Investigator: _____   .Date: _____

My signature as witness certifies that the subject signed this consent form in my presence as his/her voluntary act and deed.

Witness : _____   *Date:* _____

Appendix B
Example: photography consent document

Title of Project: Physical activity, function, muscle performance and learning in community-dwelling older adults
Principal Investigator: I. M. Keen BSc (Physio.) Postgraduate student, School of Therapy, Western University. Tel 111-2000
Tel 111-2222 (after work hours)
Project Supervisor: Dr Academe PhD. Senior Lecturer, School of Therapy, Western University. Telephone 111-2000

I. M. Keen has explained to me that photographs are required in order to illustrate various aspects of the study for the thesis and other articles, and at presentations or conferences. These images may also be converted to electronic formats for use in multi-media presentations and documents accessible to others by computer for the purpose of sharing the results of the study and for promoting this research. By giving my consent I authorize I. M. Keen and Dr Academe to use any of the photographs taken of me in printed format, in slides for presentation, and in electronic format.

Consent
I have read and understood the contents of this form and have received a copy.

Signature: _____   Date: _____
  Subject / Parent / Guardian / Custodian

I have explained to the subject how the photographs will be used, and the implications of electronic conversion and the subsequent use of images in this format, and have answered all questions.

Principal Investigator: _____   Date: _____

Appendix C
Example: subject recruitment form

Name _____   Phone _____

Introduce yourself. Describe the study, purpose and benefits. Ask if they are interested in participating.

Yes No
[1] [2] →*Thank them for taking interest in the study.*

Yes No
[1] [2] Are you 65 years or older?
                ↘ *Thank them for taking interest in the study.*

Proceed with questions

No Yes
[2] [1] Have you ever had a stroke or a heart attack?

No Yes
[2] [1] Have you ever been told you have high blood pressure?

        No Yes
        [2] [1] Do you take medication for it?

No Yes
[2] [1] Has your doctor ever told you have that you have arthritis?

        No Yes
        [2] [1] Do you have rheumatoid arthritis? (exclude myositis also)

        No Yes
        [2] [1] Do you have osteoarthritis?

        No Yes
        [2] [1] Do you have arthritis in your hips [ ] knees [ ] or ankles [ ]?

                No Yes
                [2] [1] Do you feel that this affects your ability to perform tasks requiring you to bend your knees, such as kneeling or climbing stairs?

No Yes
[2] [1] Has your doctor ever told you that you have weak bones (osteoporosis)?

If the answer to any of the above questions is YES consult the Guidelines for Subject Exclusion.

Include in the study?

No Yes
[2] [1] → *Thank them for taking interest in the study.*

Arrange an appointment
Date _____   Time _____

Assign a subject number _____

Appendix D
Example: equipment set-up check form

COMPARISON OF SINGLE AND COMBINED MANUAL HANDLING TASKS

In movement lab – video area
Plinths from centre moved to right side of room ☐
Camera 1, VCR and monitor set up and connected together ☐
Spotlight set up and connected to video trolley power board ☐

In movement lab – subject preparation area
Plinths arranged ☐
Bike in place ☐
Clean towels (2) ☐

In movement lab – handling area
Desks in place, cord taped ☐
Ballast, scoop and trolley in place ☐
Stool in place ☐

In movement lab – general
Heaters (4) on ☐
Doors closed ☐
Notice up ☐

Investigator 1
Cassettes sorted ☐
Videos sorted ☐
Forms sorted ☐

Appendix E
Principles of typography

With the advent of the computer, writers of all types of documents have been given the freedom to create their own documents with reasonable ease. However, the control that computers give over elements of typography can sometimes be counterproductive if the user is not aware of the basic principles. As a result, documents are often in danger of appearing cluttered and unbalanced. With an understanding of the principles of typography and document layout this problem can usually be avoided.

TYPEFACE
The terms typeface or font refer to a family of characters with a specific design. Despite the amazing variety of typefaces available, they can all be classified into three basic styles: serif, sans serif or script. Sans serif typefaces do not have finishing strokes at the end of the letterforms, whereas serif typefaces have short lines or curves projecting from the ends of certain letterforms. Helvetica, Arial, Geneva and **Chicago** are examples of sans serif fonts; Palatino, Times, New York, and Century Schoolbook are examples of serif fonts; **Monotype Corsiva** is a script font. Typefaces can be identified by looking for key letters T, g and M, which usually have distinctive features.

Legibility studies have found that in many situations blocks of text in serif typefaces are easier to read, the theory being that the serifs help move the eye from one letter to the next without the letters blurring together, and contribute to the recognition of individual letters. On the other hand, sans serif typefaces are generally easier to read at very large or very small sizes. Sans serif fonts are also preferred in situations where there is poor contrast between the background and the text, or when the text will be reproduced at a low resolution (e.g. using a photocopier or scanner, or computer monitor).

SIZE, WEIGHT, SLANT AND STYLE
Type is measured by its vertical height, from the top of the capital letter or ascender (whichever is higher) to the bottom of the descender (Fig. 1). The size is expressed in points, with 72 points (pt) to an inch (Fig. 2).

Typefaces can also have different weights, such as normal or bold, which refers to the density of the letters. This is determined by the width of the strokes used to make up the letters. The angle of the strokes, whether vertical or inclined, deter-

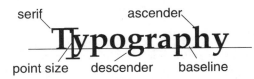

Figure 1   The anatomy of type

Figure 2   Differences in font size and typeface style

Helvetica Regular **Helvetica Bold** Palatino Regular **Palatino Bold**
roman *italic* outline shadow

Figure 3   Examples of different typefaces and typeface styles

The lines of a paragraph can be set **flush left**, flush right, centred or justified.	The lines of a paragraph can be set flush left, **flush right**, centred or justified.	The lines of a paragraph can be set flush left, flush right, **centred** or justified.	The lines of a paragraph can be set flush left, flush right, centred or **justified**.

Figure 5   Different types of paragraph alignment

Figure 4   The distinctive shapes created by upper- and lower-case letters make it easier to recognize words; words in all capitals have no variation in shape

mines the slant of the typeface. Typefaces with vertical strokes are called roman and inclined type is called italic or oblique. For computer-generated type the latter two characteristics may also be called styles, and other special effects such as outline or shadow are also available (Fig. 3).

PROVIDING EMPHASIS

Two techniques are available for providing emphasis or for improving legibility. These are typographical cueing and spatial cueing.

Typographical cueing involves the use of different typeface sizes and styles to emphasize important items (such as headings), to separate items that are not related, and to relate items that are similar (headings of the same level).

When used inappropriately, boldface, italic, underline and all capital letters (all caps) can sometimes have the opposite effect of what was intended. Boldface is generally the most effective way to make things stand out, and is therefore useful in titles and headings, or to emphasize **key words** within sentences. Too much bold can make the page look uneven and dark.

Italic type may be the most misused of all forms of emphasis: italic text is actually softer, not bolder, than normal text and it can sometimes be more difficult to read. Special styles such as shadow and outline generally should not be used for emphasis, as the letters are hollow and therefore weaker.

All capitals can be used to provide emphasis in titles but should be avoided for blocks of text. Words set in upper and lower case have distinctive and therefore easily recognizable shapes (Fig. 4). It is these shapes that are memorized when one first learns to read, and which enable one to read quickly word by word rather than letter by letter. WORDS SET IN ALL CAPS LOOK LIKE RECTANGLES OF DIFFERENT LENGTHS AND ARE MORE DIFFICULT TO READ, ESPECIALLY IN RUNNING TEXT, WHERE THERE ISN'T MUCH SPACE BETWEEN LETTERS AND LINES.

Like all caps, <u>underlining</u> is a form of emphasis inherited from the days of the typewriter, when it was difficult to change typeface size and weight. Underlining can be used to provide emphasis to headings or to specific elements within a paragraph (such as the title of a book or journal).

Type size can also be altered to provide emphasis, particularly for titles and headings. Type size generally should not exceed 24 pt for titles or headings in printed material.

Typeface styles should be used sparingly and no more than two typographical cues should be used at a time.

Spatial cueing involves the use of vertical or horizontal spacing devices, such as blank lines, indents and columns, to distinguish or relate items on a page. Generally, increased space around an item will separate it from other elements on the page, whereas decreasing the space groups items together.

The characteristics of paragraph alignment and style are made in reference to the shape of the type block relative to the margins. The lines of a paragraph can be set flush left, flush right, centred or justified (Fig. 5). Flush left is the recommended alignment for text, as it is easier to read and allows even word spacing. Pages with justified text appear neater at the margins but can have 'rivers and valleys' of white space between words (justified text is not appropriate for narrow columns).

The researching therapist should use typographical and spatial cueing with care when creating written and audiovisual materials for research communications.

Glossary

Abstract a summary placed at the beginning of a **thesis** or journal **article** which summarizes the key features of the study.

Alpha probability (Pα) chance of obtaining a difference or relationship as large as that found in the **sample,** if there is no difference or relationship between the **variables** in the whole **population**. For example, $t_{10} = 10.98$, $P = 0.02$, the chance (alpha probability) of getting a difference between two sample groups as large as that represented by a statistic of 10.98 if there was no difference in the population was 2 in 100.

Article term used to describe a published paper on research findings in a journal or newsletter.

Beta probability (Pβ) chance of being wrong if the **null hypothesis** is retained. Usually a beta probability of < 0.20 is considered acceptable. $1-β$ = **power**.

Case whether characters are capitalized or not. In upper case all characters are capitalized. In title case the first character in each word is capitalized. In sentence case the first character in the sentence in capitalized. In lower case no characters are capitalized.

Clinical significance the extent to which the findings of a study are clinically meaningful or relevant.

Critical alpha probability **alpha probability** below which the **null hypothesis** would be rejected and the **research hypothesis** accepted. Commonly 0.01, 0.05 or 0.10 depending on the precision of the measurement.

Data a set of facts or figures collected during a research study.

Datum a single bit of information.

Dependent variable the variable in the **research hypothesis** which changes as a result of manipulation of the **independent variable**. Otherwise known as the response variable.

Dissertation see **thesis**.

Empirical based on data rather than opinion, tradition or hearsay. Usually data considered to be from research, that is, a systematic investigation rather than coincidental or casual observation which is termed anecdotal evidence.

Exclusion criteria a set of characteristics which an individual must not have in order to be included in the **population** of a study. Usually characteristics which are thought likely to put the **subject** in unacceptable risk or cost if they participate or interfere with the quality of the data or the interpretation of the findings.

Extraneous variable a variable that may affect the relationship between the **independent** and the **dependent variables**. Also known as confounding variable.

Figure refers to all illustrative material (e.g. diagrams, graphs, photographs) in a research communication which are not tables or text.

Footnote a phrase or sentence placed below the body of text, table or figure which provides additional information validating or clarifying a point, statement or argument.

Guiding question a question stating what the researcher is trying to find out. Used where a **hypothesis** is not appropriate.

Hypothesis a statement of the expected relationship between variables which can be statistically tested.

Inclusion criteria a set of characteristics which an individual must have to be included in the population of a study.

Independent variable the variable in the research hypothesis which is manipulated so that the effect on the **dependent variable** can be observed.

Literature review the summaries and critical analyses of the literature relating to the topic of the research or research question.

Manuscript a research report submitted to a journal for publication.

Materials the equipment, instruments or measurement tools used in a study.

Null hypothesis (H_0) a statement that there is no difference or relationship between variables. In classical western science, experiments are designed to falsify the null hypothesis, leaving the only sensible explanation to be the **research hypothesis**.

Operational definition the definition of a variable

which states how the variable will be used in a particular study, for example the procedures involved when measuring a **dependent variable** or how an **independent variable** will be manipulated.

Participants the individuals who take part in a study. In qualitative research this term tends to be used in preference to 'subjects' and sometimes includes the researcher as well.

Pilot study a study carried out prior to the main study with the aim of highlighting and resolving data collection and analysis problems.

Population (N) all who meet **inclusion criteria** but not **exclusion criteria**.

Power ability of a study or statistical test to detect a difference or relationship in the data collected from a sample. Power can be increased by increasing sample size, increasing effect size or decreasing measurement error. Usually power > 0.80 is considered acceptable. Power = $1-\beta$.

Probability (P) the likelihood or chance of an event occurring. Usually represented as P and a number between 0 (never occurs) and 1 (certain to occur), e.g. $P = 0.04$

Qualitative research research based on the analysis of data which is not represented as numbers. Qualitative research methods tend to have a holistic philosophical view which encourages investigation of subjective experiences of individuals within their social context. Examples include ethnography, phenomenology, action research and grounded theory.

Quantitative research research based on the analysis of data which is represented as numbers. Quantitative research methods tend to have a mechanistic and deterministic philosophical view which encourages the reduction of problems to the investigation of variables which can be measured objectively. Examples include randomized controlled trials, repeated measures, factorial, experimental and small n/time series analysis.

Research proposal a document outlining a planned project or investigation. The research proposal includes the background to the problem to be investigated, the **research hypotheses/guiding questions** and procedures for data collection and analysis.

Research hypothesis (H_A) a statement which predicts the expected outcome of a study. Also known as the alternative hypothesis as it is the one retained when **the null hypothesis** has been rejected. When there are multiple research hypotheses they are commonly denoted H_1, H_2, etc.

Sample (n) the subgroup of a **population** who are actually recruited to a study.

Statistical significance demonstration that the result obtained is unlikely to be due to chance. Usually when **alpha probability** is below 0.01, 0.05 or 0.10.

Subjects the individuals from whom information is collected for a study (e.g. therapists, patients, healthy individuals).

Thesis a detailed discourse on a subject. Terms thesis and **dissertation** are used differently in different countries.

Type I error when the **null hypothesis** is rejected and **research hypothesis** accepted based on **sample** data, when the null hypothesis is true for the **population**. Chance of Type I error is **alpha probability**.

Type II error when the **null hypothesis** is retained (and **research hypothesis** not accepted) based on **sample** data, when the research hypothesis is true for the **population**. Chance of a Type II error is **beta probability**.

Variable a characteristic that can be measured, observed or manipulated and that can take on different values either quantitatively or qualitatively.

Withdrawal criteria a set of characteristics which would result in the withdrawal of a subject after they were included. Withdrawal is usually due to failure of the subject to participate or where the subject status changes such that the subject may be at unacceptable risk or cost to continue or where their data may be of poor quality.

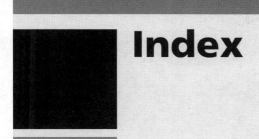

Index

Numbers in bold refer to tables and illustrations; numbers followed by the letter 'g' refer to glossary entries